To, Pete Masterson
from District Govern

ALMOST TO HEAVEN

ALMOST TO HEAVEN

The 40-year History of the Texas Lions Camp for Crippled Children

By Mary Mae Hartley

FIRST EDITION

Printed in the United States of America
By Nortex Press
A Division of Eakin Publications, Inc., Austin, Texas

PHOTO CREDITS

Ron Anderson	Jayne Schulte
Roy Ortiz	Rand Southard
Judy Anderson	Andrea Dunn
David Thomas	Glenn Crawford

COVER PHOTO by Ron Anderson, Director of Development and Public Relations for the Texas Lions Camp.

Contents

Introduction vii
1 The Quest Began When Polio Raged 1
2 Traveling Salesmen 16
3 That First Summer 26
4 Boundless Imagination and Twenty-Four-Hour Duty 35
5 A New World 49
6 The Invisible Disease 60
7 Keys to Camping: The Counselors 74
8 Mother Nature's Classroom 88
9 Let This Horse Do My Walking 98
10 Camp Tailtwisters 105
11 A Lion Never Rests 122
12 It Takes Many Hearts 131
13 Grassroots of the Camp: The Staff 140
14 White Cane Club 150
15 The Doors Never Close 158
Epilogue 181

Acknowledgment

Texas Lions League Board of Directors join me in expressing appreciation for the support, hard work, and encouragement given the Texas Lions Camp. You and those who came before have established a living legacy through the lives of children with disabilities. A child with a disability has a great desire to be like all other children. You have given that opportunity to thousands by allowing them to learn about themselves, develop their innate abilities, and give them hope for the future.

We regret that every person, Lion, Lioness, business, and foundation who have assisted the Camp cannot be named. It certainly does not diminish each contribution. The vital services provided handicapped children cannot be done without you. Herb Petry, past president of the International Association of Lions Clubs, said, "Some who give and do the most are not always recognized. The Camp became an organization of everyday people believing in a dream. They wanted to be part of a group that was doing something for unfortunate children." The chance to realize that dream continues.

Glenn Crawford
Executive Director
Texas Lions League for
Crippled Children, Inc.

Introduction

Summer had not come down full force in all her brightness and heat as yet, so the June breezes played in the tall grasses. They brushed through the leaves of the giant oaks, which leaned from years of combatting the rough Texas Hill Country. A skinny, bent figure slowly plodded up the path to the most "mystical" place for all the camper-children. They called it just what it was, Inspiration Point.

Robbie *had* to make it to the top. He *had* to prove to himself he could. He thought of the muscles he had built up during his stay at camp, and the challenges that pushed him to his physical capacity. He had done things at camp which a crippled boy never dreamed possible!

Following him at some distance were his unit leader and a counselor. They lagged behind because Robbie had insisted he needed to do this on his own to prove something to himself. Robbie guessed that it already had been about two hours.

Somehow, if he got to the top of Inspiration Point — alone, on his own — Robbie knew he would find the sense of freedom that his twisted legs had always ached to find. Then everyone else would know, too. His life would change, not that it hadn't already at camp.

His crutches crunched into the loose gravel of the path, long worn by others like him striving so hard to reach that top. Crunch, crunch. It was slow going for the boy and was scary at times, too. The rubber cap on one crutch had been scraped off, and Robbie's arms, strong from supporting his whole body the past twelve years, were beginning to feel tired. But he would make it! Sweat trickled down his cheeks, red from the extra exertion. He managed a smile as a jack rabbit scurried from the underbrush and stopped a few feet away, watching the boy's progress. Robbie had learned a lot about animals at this children's camp.

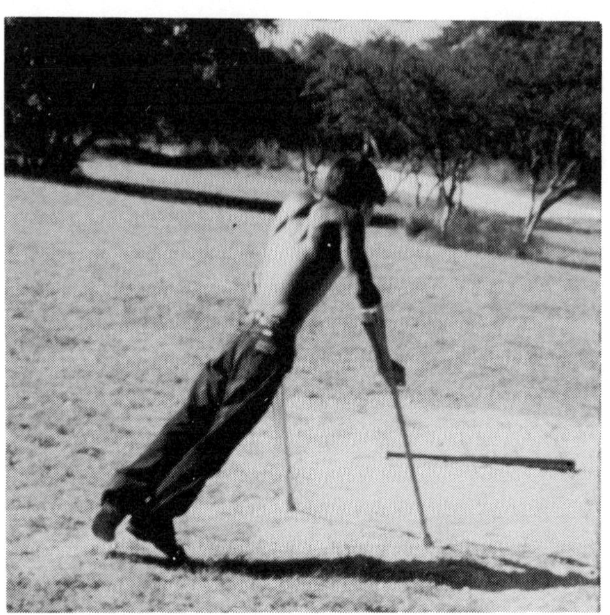

Hiking the hard way, but it built muscles.

Twice on the way up Robbie had fallen. Back home, parent's hands would have quickly picked him up and placed him on his crutches, but he was on his own here. It reminded him of the day before when little Jackson was struggling to hold his tray of food in the dining hall, while maneuvering slowly on his walker. He had fallen. Food scattered everywhere. Jackson had sprawled on the floor. Not one of the campers or counselors in the dining hall moved. Jackson worked hard, using his torso to painfully back up against a wall where he could, with the help of his hands, pull himself and his useless legs far enough to grab hold of the walker. He was up once more!

At that special moment all 350 kids and counselors stood up and cheered! It had been an unexpected triumph for little Jackson. Now Robbie would have his own triumph. He was nearing the top of the hill. His breath was almost gone, but his resolution held firm. The crutches kept slowly moving, one side, then the other side. Crunch, crunch. Just a few more feet.

Then, with one more crunchy slide, he reached the top! "I'm superman," he thought between gasps of breath, and his arms began trembling. Robbie rested the tired arms on the pads of his now still wooden "legs." The purple hills were below him; and across the valley, he saw Kerrville in the distance. Above him were blue skies. "It's like being almost to Heaven," he whispered to himself. He looked down at the crutches which would always be his companions, but no longer his captors. He began laughing. From now on, he would keep laughing, in spite of his handicaps. Boy, what would they think at home? He hoped they would be proud of him.

He looked back down the path. There came the two major supporters of his significant effort. They were yelling and wildly making the victory sign. Now he could hear them, as they, too, panted up the last few feet of path. "You did it, Robbie! You did it!" They grabbed him and hugged him. This was what the camp called a "group hug." It was also called "love and caring." Robbie let loose and turned to look again over the expanse of hazy blue hills in the distance and vivid green fields below.

One of the counselors was remembering a few summers back when several older campers in wheelchairs decided they would make the long climb to Inspiration Point in their wheelchairs traveling on the little used back path which was filled with sharp rocks and deep ruts and which was much rougher than the one Robbie just climbed. They made it, and it was the talk of the whole camp that summer. Parents at home heard about the heroes of the camp. It was no more a triumph than Robbie had just won. The counselors knew that all the other boys and girls at camp would be waiting for the newest hero; they were sure each one had some fingers crossed for Robbie.

At this moment several hundred miles away, along the Texas-Mexico border in Brownsville, sat a graying, elderly man smiling to himself. As usual, he was remembering those beautiful children that he had seen do almost impossible things at the Texas Lions Camp. For some of them the most important thing they learned was how to get in and out of their wheelchairs alone. For others it marked a personal success to be able to lace their shoes, even though they could not see them.

Jack Wiech, the first president of the Texas Lions League, and hundreds of his fellow Lions Club members in Texas had dedicated their service careers to the crippled children who had no camp available for summer fun or for rehabilitation. "We will build a

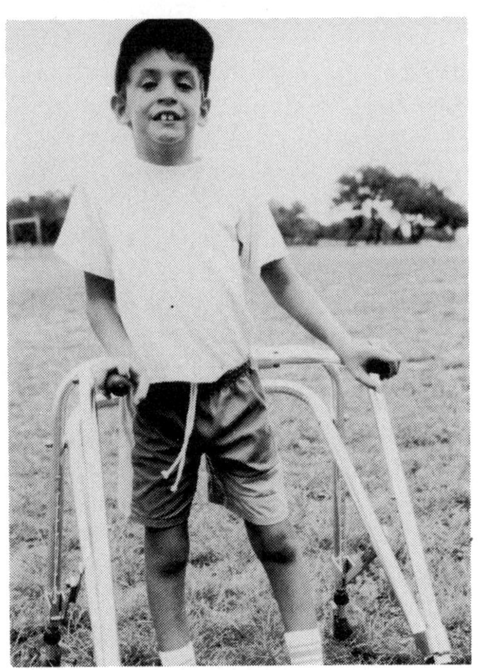

Kids breathed better in the outdoors.

camp where they can go, and grow, and learn, and experience new adventures. They will be able to forget afflictions and will develop skills," the Lions promised. They kept those promises. Never in all those forty years since 1949 had their dream wavered. Each year brought new challenges, which were met.

There was a special trait of Lions Clubs members: when they began a project, they did it right! They thought big! So, in Texas, they founded the best crippled children's camp anywhere in the world. Year after year they continued the battle for their special children and their special camp.

On Robbie's triumphal day at Inspiration Point, Wiech was thinking of Lions like Jack Roe, whose idea of a camp for handicapped children was the basis for the Texas Lions project. He also recalled the work of League founders, like J. I. Moore, Reagan Smith, and Virgil Minear. What a blessing their idea had been!

Back at the camp near Kerrville was nine-year-old Jennifer, who had been blind since birth and who had one arm missing. She perched on the edge of a diving board above the deep end of the swimming pool, and her one thin arm bent just right so that she

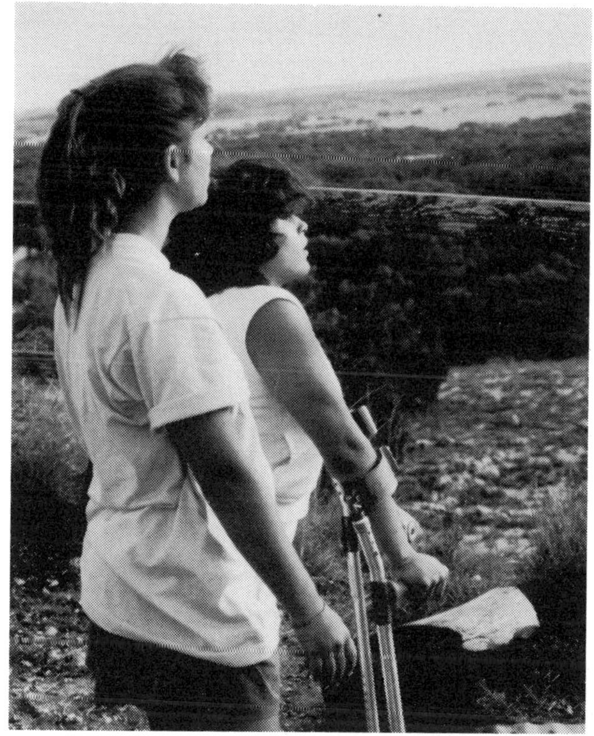

Inspiration Point was for dreaming.

lurched forward in the air, diving quite skillfully into the friendly waters. She swam on the bottom of the pool, then made her way to the top and reached the ladder at the side. Her courage had given her a new lease on life. She was beginning to realize that she, too, could take charge of her young life. At the Lions League Camp she was taught to "see" things she had never seen before. A wonderland had opened to her, and she was the Alice. Jennifer was as happy with herself as were Robbie and little Jackson.

Jack Wiech felt confident that when he was gone, other Lions would carry on the work of the camp. During those first four decades, Texas Lions knew that the Robbies could make it to the top of Inspiration Point, that the Jennifers could win swimming trophies, and the little Jacksons would feel they could handle themselves in spite of their disabilities. This was the basic reason for the camp.

All the children needed was a chance. Texas Lions and their friends footed the bill for forty years, providing a camp for over 40,000 boys and girls. The spirit from the very beginning of the project, for both Lions and campers, had been: ***"I can!"*** At this unique camp crippled boys and girls sprouted wings, blind children saw wonderful things and the deaf and mute heard the lovely music of the outdoors. All of the campers gained that happy promise that, after all, their lives could be lived well in spite of their physical shackles.

This was Lionism in action, and Lionism at its best.

This is the story of a dream that became a reality. It is a tribute to the lion-hearted men and women who cared enough to assure thousands of special children a bit of happiness they so desperately needed. This is the tale of one of the most enchanted camps in the world that never closes its door, and where children can reach ***almost to heaven!***

— Chapter 1 —

"The Quest Began When Polio Raged"

"No child should be denied camping just because he is crippled."
— Jack Roe

Stephen, age eleven, accompanied by his mother, appeared in the office of the YMCA and asked to register for the swimming classes. He was told he did not qualify. The mother who had seen that disappointed look in his eyes many times before, thought how unfair it was. It wasn't Stephen's fault that polio had crippled both legs. He didn't want to be this way. He was turned away, sad as usual.

Tommy, age eight, had watched his two older brothers pack and go to Boy Scout camp for as long as he could remember, and he remembered wistfully. Through a birth defect, one of his legs was four inches shorter than the other and he only had one arm. It never occurred to him that he could go to camp, too, have fun and ride a horse.

It occurred to some Texas Lions Club members in 1947 before Dr. Salk discovered the polio vaccine, when the dread disease was ravaging Texas children.

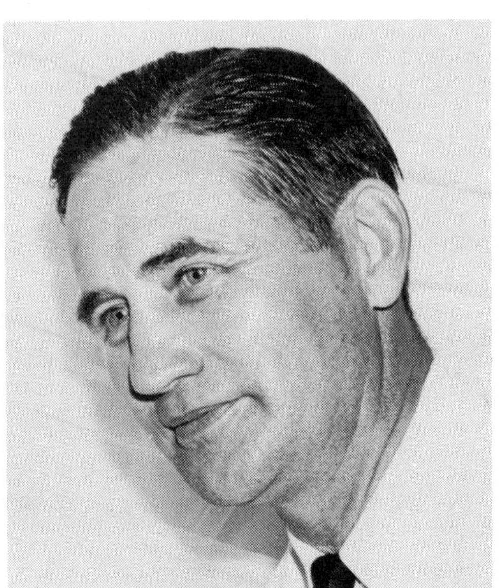
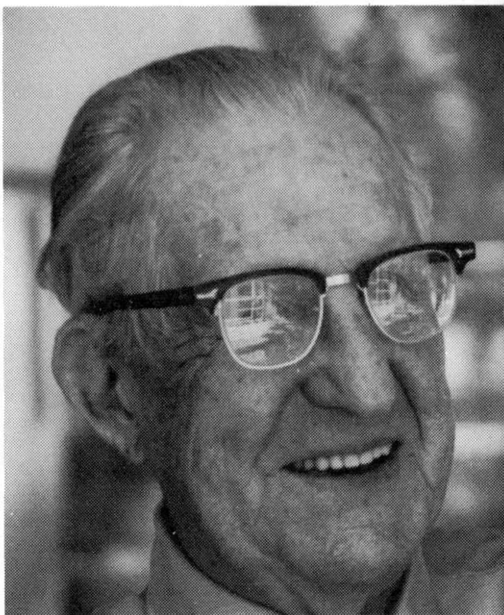

Jack Roe, left; a crippled children's camp was his idea. . . . J. I. Moore, right, one of the founders in 1949.

Characteristic of Lions members was the sharing of their visions with other Lions. They envisioned a camp for crippled children. As a result, in June of 1953 Tommy and Stephen were welcomed to the Texas Lions League Camp for Crippled Children, along with 234 other handicapped boys and girls.

The idea of a crippled children's camp was generally attributed to Jack Roe, who had been in social work and had directed YMCA recreational facilities and several camps for boys and girls. Some said it was he who planted the seed in the minds of his brothers of the Kerrville Lions Club. They said Roe convinced Jack Wiech, newly elected Governor of Lions District 2A, that camping should not be denied any children just because they were handicapped.

J. I. Moore of Kerrville, a founder of the League and lifetime member of the camp's Board of Directors, said that "if it had not been for Jack Roe there would be no Lions Camp for children. That camp needs to have a memorial built to honor Roe." Then he added, "he worked us to death to get that camp started."

Roe had moved to the Hill Country with thoughts of beginning a camp for crippled children at a small ranch he owned. At first he thought it should be a day camp, but he saw it could be done on a larger scale and encouraged the Lions Club of Kerrville to help. Roe kept talking about the camp and studying the possibilities. When the Lions League was trying to acquire the campsite from the federal government, Roe was secretary of the Kerrville Lions Club. Moore was president and later became recording secretary. Roe, Moore, and Wiech were a hard-working trio through every step of acquiring the land and setting up the camp for operation.

One historian of the children's camp described in detail how Roe and Wiech spent untold hours and much of their own money contacting Lions Clubs over Texas and conferring with persons knowledgeable in rehabilitation of handicapped children and in camping. He recounted that Roe and another Kerrville Lions club member, the Rev. Tom Brabham of the First Methodist Church, drove to the Lions Clubs International convention in New York City in 1949, presented the idea, and received their endorsement.

Lions in Texas saw the camp as a symbol of unity for them throughout the state. According to Lion Julien C. Hyer's book on the first fifty years of Lionism in Texas: "The true history of Texas Lionism is written in the lives of the thousands of crippled children served at the Lions Camp in Kerrville, in the light of hope struck in the dark of blindness by the Lions of Texas."

On September 11, 1948 the Kerrville Lions Club invited district governors to meet with them regarding the camp idea. At this meeting, Wiech expressed the view that his district would undertake the project alone, if it could not be established as the first statewide project of Texas Lions. No decisions were reached at that meeting, but the idea was firmly planted and some had seen the vision. They liked what they saw.

Other meetings followed in Texas, some informal and some organized. The leaders, mostly at their own expense, traveled the country gaining background information necessary to build such a facility. They discussed the possibilities of the camp with the Texas Departments of Public Welfare, Rehabilitation and Health. They met with orthopedic physicians and therapists and visited some twenty-eight programs dealing with crippled children located throughout the U.S. and Canada. They obtained an overall view and many ideas regarding the size of such a camp, the capital requirements, cost of operation, rehabilitation value, approximate number of potential enrollees, recommended architecture and layout of such a facility, and many other details. The Lions who were leaders in the camp project movement were prepared; they had done their homework.

After committee meetings, speeches and gatherings over the state, on March 12, 1949, the Texas Lions League for Crippled Children, Incorporated, was organized in Brownsville during a meeting of the Council of Governors of Texas. Signing the charter were Wiech, Reagan Smith of Conroe, Virgil Minear of Hallettsville, Moore, W. R. Rutherford of Dumas, Schley Riley of Big Springs and Pat Jackson of Nacogdoches. Of these men, the only surviving founders in 1989 were Wiech and Moore.

Named charter officers of the League were Wiech, president; Jackson, first vice president; Rutherford, second vice president; Minear, third vice president; Moore, recording secretary; Smith, treasurer; and Riley, financial secretary. They decided, at the first, to name the camp after Melvin Jones of Chicago, founder of Lions Clubs International. He was living at that time and asked his name to be omitted since it was a Texas-only project. So it was named Texas Lions Camp for Crippled Children. By 1989 it was generally called the Texas Lions Camp, and it was in operation on a year-round basis with many varied programs. Its most visible image throughout its history has been the summer camp for children with physical disabilities.

A month after the League was formed, the Texas Secretary of State signed a document incorporating the League as a nonprofit, tax-exempt organization. State endorsement came at the Texas Lions convention in May 1949 at San Angelo. Two months later at the annual meeting of the International Association of Lions Clubs in New York City the group approved the camp idea and voted permission for the League to use the Lions Club symbol. The ball was rolling.

District Governors of Texas agreed on several basics for establishment. First, the camp would be built and supported by the voluntary assistance of Lions and Lions Clubs of Texas and their friends; second, no charge would be made for any child admitted to the camp; third, the camp would be governed by a board of directors composed of the district governors of Texas and the camp would be managed by an executive board appointed by the board of directors.

The size of the board has been enlarged over the years to consist of the original charter members of the League, all district governors, all immediate past district governors, members of the executive committee, all past presidents of the League who remained active in the work of the League, and two members elected from each district in the state. This meant that the board grew to seventy members, over ten times as large as the original board in 1949.

The first hurdles had been cleared. Now came the big one; a suitable location for the camp. A large number of Lions turned their thoughts toward Kerrville, where the idea originated and which already was a widely recognized tourist magnet and summer camp mecca. The climate was healthful and living was easy. Over thirty private camps catering to youngsters already dotted the Hill Country around Kerrville. None, of course, were opened to crippled children. But that was soon to be corrected. Lions over the state asked the Kerrville club to search for an appropriate site. There are many stories about who first sighted the perfect spot. Somehow it filtered down to the League that there was a very nice parcel of land attached to the veterans hospital acreage just to the east of Kerrville. There was a possibility it might be classified as "surplus federal property," thus being available on a grant basis.

To Wiech and others who investigated the property, it looked wonderful. There it stood, 504 enchanted acres, a natural wildlife refuge with hills and valleys, natural springs and a view of the Guadalupe River. They envisioned this as the very special place for crippled boys and girls of Texas to have a camp of their own. This was where, without charge, kids could frolic or wheel at their own pace, in a friendly atmosphere of sharing and helping.

Originally owned by Kerrville founder Joshua Brown, this parcel of land had been given to the American Legion by the Schreiner family of Kerrville after World War I. The VA hospital said they did not plan to use the 504 acres. It was like a dream come true for the League and the Lions of Texas.

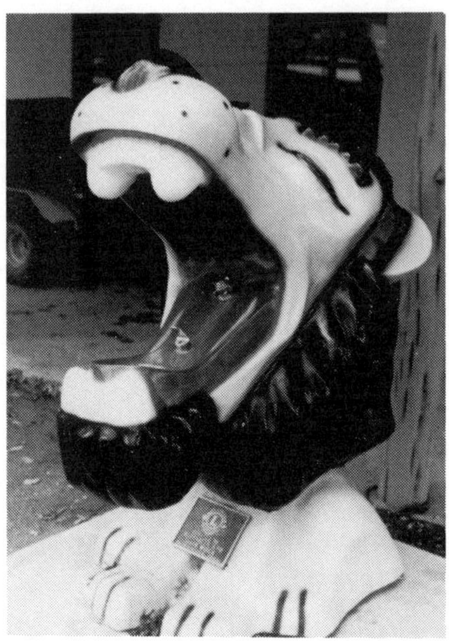

Drinking fountain on Lions campsite.

The dream soon exploded into a nightmare of governmental red tape. It was touch-and-go for a while, but there were a lot of people who cared enough to help. For some it was a real sacrifice, but it was important, these people felt. Sid Harris, noted as the Kerrville Lions Club's all-time champion ticket seller for fund-raisers, said at this time that his store was having some financial problems. Nonetheless, he and his wife, Dot, felt the camp project was so important that they borrowed money to help send representatives to Washington, D.C., to settle the land deal. At Kerrville's charity ball in 1988, Harris donated a family heirloom watch encrusted with 200 diamonds to be auctioned, with proceeds going to the camp.

The Lions network for obtaining this site operated like this: Wiech stayed in Brownsville and wrote letters and served as liaison between the state government, federal government, important backers and Bill Mickelsen. Bill, president of the Kerrville Lions Club and an architect, became the lobbyist in the nation's capitol. Almost every governmental agency in Washington, D.C. seemed to have a part in the act. It just looked that way to Mickelson and

Wiech. Looking back it seems incredible how these men, especially attorney Wiech and architect Mickelsen, could have run their own businesses during those harried months of work and worry. Did they put themselves on the back burner? Any Lion in Texas will answer, "Yes."

It was necessary to understand Lionism and its *one* purpose, in order to understand such men as Wiech, Roe, and Mickelson. The worldwide motto for the Lions organization, sometimes seen on caps, jackets, pins and banners, was composed of two words: "*we serve.*" Unless a person was dedicated to service, there was no need to join a Lions club. Their code of ethics said: ". . . to aid . . . my fellowmen . . . by giving my sympathy to those in distress . . . my aid to the weak . . . and my substance . . . to the needy." This code was visible in 1947 when the Lions service was directed to the many children crippled by polio. Boys and girls were spending their young years in and out of iron lungs and struggling to walk in cumbersome braces. Their needs were overwhelming. Lions Club members did not meet socially, although they had great fun together in their projects. They met to consider how best they could help those in need, then they gave their own money, time, and energy in support of their selected project. That was Lionism.

Marshall Cooper, League president in 1987–88, wrote in his column in the camp newspaper, that unless one had driven a crippled child, who is a little scared and very apprehensive, to camp at Kerrville, then returned in two weeks to find a happy and confident camper; unless one had sat down with a curly-headed little girl who didn't understand what had happened to her body, and had attempted to explain how diabetes can cut her life expectancy by at least one-third and why she needed daily insulin shots; unless one had seen a camper gyrate his wheelchair to a western band tune; unless one had walked in these small moccasins

. . . it would be hard to understand the compelling reason men and women throughout Texas so dearly loved *their* Lions camp and so enthusiastically had met the challenge, year after year, of never closing the doors to any of *their* children.

The children's camp was to become a symbol of Texas Lionism, and its supporters expected it to keep blossoming, reaching out and enfolding the many handicapped children who so desperately clung to the big Lion hands. It gave them hope. Hope was what kept the original workers going strong in 1949 and 1950. Among the first officials contacted by Texas Lions Secretary Marlowe C. Fisher was Dr. George Cox, head of the Texas Health Department, who became a staunch ally. Dr. Cox first wrote to Texas Congressman O. C. Fisher and Senator Lyndon Johnson, explaining to them what the Texas Lions Clubs proposed to do, and why they wanted that beautiful piece of land near Kerrville. He thought they would be influential persons to help convince the federal government to grant the land to the Lions League.

Meanwhile, Wiech corresponded with the Federal Security Agency's field representative, F. A. Ramsey, in Dallas. The FSA was the guardian of surplus government property. About this time, the League discovered the land was about to be sold to a private firm for development. It took some behind-the-scenes work in Washington to get this deal cancelled, so that first opportunity could go to the nonprofit, rehabilitation and recreational facility planned by the Lions. This was successful, but red tape was still to be encountered.

Dr. Cox wrote also to the regional director of the U.S. Public Health Service, advising him of the Lions League's desire for the property. He outlined all details of the proposed camp project, which the League had painstakingly put together. They knew all agencies would need the entire focus of the project in order to make a decision. At first, officials seemed to think that the only way for the Lions to obtain the property was for the federal government to deed it to the Texas state government which, in turn, could relinquish its rights to the Lions of Texas. This was one reason Dr. Cox had assumed a position in the negotiations. The other reason was that he realized the great need for such a camp. The state had nothing like it for rehabilitation and recreation of children with disabilities.

Mickelsen had been visiting with Senator Johnson's chief assistant, John Connally, in Washington, D.C. Some questions raised were: can the League justify a request for all the 504 acres; can they show an immediate or future need for that much of the land; can they operate the project just as well with less acreage?

A new analysis was prepared by Mickelsen in which he out-

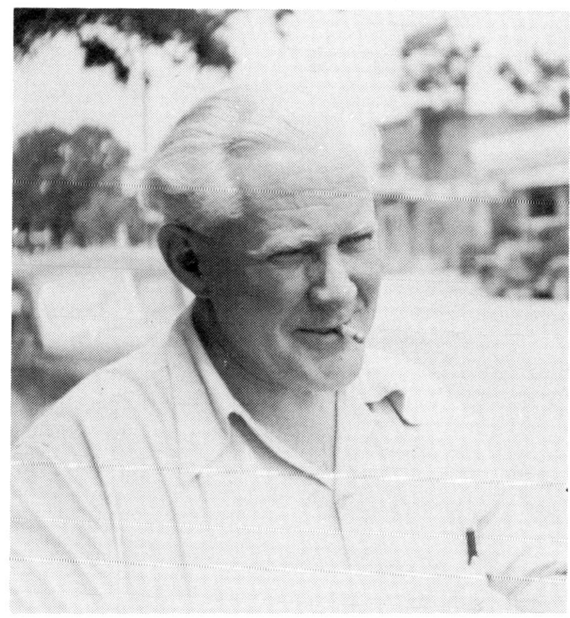

Bill Mickelsen, architect for the camp, whose spirit would always keep watch.

lined the following desirable aspects of this particular tract: With over 22,000 crippled children in the state, the 504 acres would be needed for expansion; public utilities were within easy reach of the site; surface drainage proved there was practically no sign of storm water erosion; the tract had access to hospitals in case of medical emergencies; the Guadalupe River on the southwest boundary would make boating, fishing, and other water sports close at hand; a large state park was directly across the river and use of its trails, roads, and picnic areas would be an added bonus to campers and families; the natural terrain afforded excellent places for athletic fields, staff housing development, hiking trails, and trails for horse and pony carts. In general, the land was very conducive to a camp for children.

Wiech kept up a constant correspondence with Senator Johnson's office and many other D.C. contacts, for the urgency remained. The Lions must get the land grant before anyone else. He wrote LBJ: "The Lions of Texas decided that no more worthwhile statewide project could be undertaken by our organization than the establishment, maintenance and operation of a crippled children's camp where all crippled children of Texas would have the opportunity to come, without charge, and receive supervised rehabilitation training. Unquestionably the need for such facilities in Texas is great, yet there is not a single crippled children's camp in the state at this time."

Prominent men about the state, whether a Lions member or not, wrote letters in behalf of the project. San Antonio Attorney Adrian A. Spears wrote his friend Senator Johnson, saying that he knew the Senator would help as much as he could on this idea but he just wanted him to know that he would personally appreciate anything that the Senator could do. He told LBJ that he knew the many thousands of Lions throughout Texas would also appreciate his help.

Weeks went tediously by. Wiech received a long letter from Congressman Fisher explaining that a new piece of legislation was before the Senate at that time, having passed the House of Representatives, that would change prospectives and make acquisition of federal surplus land easier.

After a meeting in Kerrville between Congressman Fisher, Mickelsen, Roe and Kerrville Lion George Brown, Mickelsen went on several missions to the nation's capitol. While there Congressman Fisher, who completely supported the camp idea, invited Mickelsen to make his headquarters at his office. He also put the Texas Lions representative in touch with the right people.

One of Mickelsen's three-day stays in Washington went something like this: he reiterated all details of the proposed camp in Congressman Fisher's office; met with R. G. Church at the Office of Surplus Real Estate, Public Building Administration; had dinner with Mr. Church; another appointment with Fisher; met with a Mr. Beaser, general counsel for Children's Division, Federal Security Administration; a meeting with John Connally; talked with Arthur C. Perry in Senator Tom Connally's office; lunch with Mr. Church; meeting with Mr. Beaser and two attorneys from FSA; back to Fisher's office to report progress; talked on telephone with George Brown and George Gentry of Austin regarding an appointment in the U.S. Attorney General's office which had been made for Mickelsen by Texas Lieutenant Governor Allan Shivers; talked with A. D. Vansch, then J. E. Williams in Attorney General's office, then the General himself, Tom Clark, who assured Mickelsen of his complete cooperation with the project. Back to Fisher's office he reported that the General indicated when House Bill 4754 and Senate Bill 2020 passed, he thought the Lions should readily qualify for a grant under the provisions of these bills and the federal government could deed the property to the League.

It wasn't over yet. There was much paperwork to be done. On November 1, 1949, Mickelsen wrote Wiech that "The meat of what I have to report is that we now have definite assurances from every agency or departmental authority in Washington that the 504 acres we request for our camp site will become Texas Lions League for Crippled Children property at 100 percent discount, subject to stipulated use and occupancy in conformity with our stated intent."

Mickelsen went home to Kerrville, but soon returned to D.C. to file applications. He learned that a field inspection of the property had been done by the Federal Security Agency. Then, at last, the legislation passed both Congress and Senate which made acquisition of the Kerrville land possible for the League. Said Mickelsen to Wiech: "I found every individual unreservedly receptive to our project aims and warmly inclined to push ahead as rapidly as possible. They *did* push other matters aside and concentrated upon our application."

About this time the Texas Lions governors council met in Kerrville and toured the site that they had almost acquired. And one of the state's most prestigious Lions, Herb Petry of Carrizo Springs who was the youngest president ever to serve Lions Clubs International, changed his mind about the camp project and lent his forceful support. Petry originally opposed the camp idea because the League proposed to support it by taking a portion of all Lions dues and giving it to the camp operation. He began pointing with pride to this camp as the best example of "Lionism in Action," all over the world.

He was quoted in the Hyer book years later: "I shall never forget the meeting in Carrizo Springs during those early formative years when Jack Wiech, the first camp president, came to see me with some Kerrville Lions and several of the district governors. I should never have questioned the vision of the Lions of Texas and their courage to make their dreams a reality. No, I shouldn't have because today we have near Kerrville, Texas, an outstanding project that belongs to all of the Lions of Texas. Each year it is touching the lives of almost 1,000 handicapped people in our state and giving to these less fortunate people encouragement and inspiration to face the challenges of life, though handicapped. Certainly, what is being done in Kerrville under the banner of Texas Lionism must be pleasing in the sight of Him who first taught us to serve, to be our brother's keeper, and to put the Golden Rule into practice."

The first of 1950 brought news from the Federal Security Agency that the request for the land application was "legally insufficient." More information was needed. The League had thought that every single bit of information that could possibly be squeezed out, had been! A new name appeared in correspondence, a new cog in the Washington machine, and he needed all information plus additional application. The League complied.

Finally, on August 1, 1950, after over a year of constant work, the sale of agreement was signed in the Dallas office of the Federal Security Administrator. Officials in Washington who signed the sales agreement were the director of the Division of School Administration; chief of Surplus Property Utilization Program; head of the Real Property Disposal of the General Services; general counsel for General Services; U.S. Commissioner of Education; and the Administrator of General Services. Signing for the League was its president, Jack Wiech.

The League sent out news over Texas that the first step toward founding their proposed camp was complete. It reminded Lion members, friends, and the general public that what the League hoped to do was to provide a beautiful camping service for as many Texas crippled children as possible. President Wiech added that this dream would be able to grow with the acquired 504 acres, where the League would build and then keep expanding to help more and more children.

Senator Lyndon Johnson had written many letters keeping Wiech and the League informed of activities in the nation's capitol on behalf of the Lions' request for the surplus land. The future President of the United States sent telegrams stating "delighted to tell you Federal Security Agency and General Services Administration have approved transfer of land near Legion for crippled children's program of Texas Lions League." Another indicated he would be happy to be of service to them at any time in the future. He also was disappointed he could not attend the formal groundbreaking in 1950 and camp dedication services in 1953.

The 504 enchanted acres now belonged to the Texas Lions League for Crippled Children, Incorporated. But not without strings! One provision required the League to raise $100,000 in six months to guarantee construction of the proposed nonprofit rehabilitation camp. So the League began an uphill battle to secure that $100,000. At first, only eight percent of the Lions in Texas had taken a financial interest in the camp idea. Supporters were finding that sometimes dreams were hard to sell.

First, the League devised a Life Membership status for Lions, under which one paid $100 and became a member for life and received a gold certificate. Later they designed a golden pin to be worn next to the heart of the life members. This brought in some money, and next they planned a statewide fund drive. To launch the drive, a radio broadcast in Austin featured Texas Governor Allan Shivers, a Lion himself. Other speakers on that memorable radio program were League President Wiech and past International Lions Clubs President Petry. These men's voice went into every corner of the state loud and clear. It was a rousing beginning.

Next, the League considered employing a professional fundraiser; but in a bold move one day, the League directors decided to take the project directly to the clubs of Texas in a face-to-face campaign. This took manpower, time, and energy. A lot of Lions met with a lot of other Lions over the state. Wiech was on a continuous speaking tour. His first meeting was with the Downtown Dallas Lions Club. The League thought that if they could sell this club on the camp idea, others in the state would follow. It was in Dallas a generation earlier that Lions Clubs International had been born.

To help make selling easier, Mickelsen designed a large, detailed scale model of the proposed camp, and J. C. "Buddy" Murray, a Kerrville Lion who was a longtime maintenance supervisor at the camp, built it. The model showed hills, valleys, buildings, and playgrounds. It was impressive. Wiech carted it all over the state in the back of his station wagon, trying to raise the necessary $100,000.

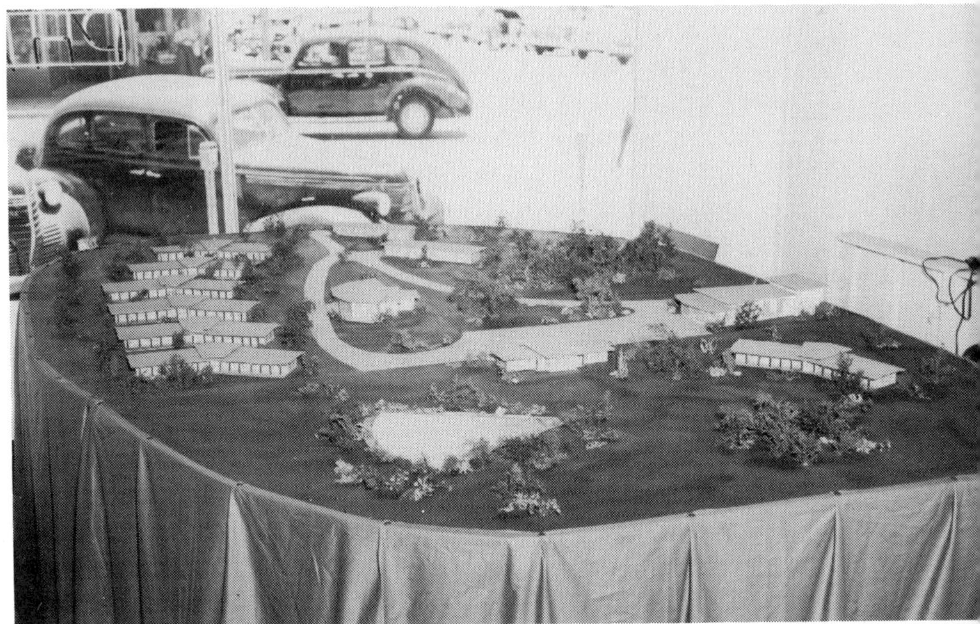

Model of the camp which convinced Texas Lions to unite and create their dream for handicapped children.

At that first Dallas presentation he pointed out to the Lions that no child ever asked to be admitted into this world; that a child was handicapped through no fault of his own; that despite handicaps, every child had the right to a happy childhood full of fun and learning and growing as an important human being. He was eloquent and appealing; he spoke from the heart and he spoke to the heart. When his Dallas talk ended, one of the most vigorous opponents of the camp idea became a life member on the spot. Lion George R. Jordan, a past international president, explained he had fought the idea at first because he thought it would duplicate such good projects as the Shrine's Crippled Children's Hospital. He realized that the project proposed was a camp, not a hospital. Soon the only two Texas Lions District Governors who opposed the camp also crossed over the line and became supporters.

Even with the success in Dallas, then over the state, trouble loomed on the horizon. The six months required for raising the $100,000 was drawing to a close, and the money goal was about $20,000 short. During the march for funds, the hard-working Lions had discovered two important things: they could do the job themselves, and the camp was proving to be a unifying project for Texas Lions.

Down to the finish line came the League, wondering where they could get the last $20,000. They had tapped all possible sources for the needed funds, they thought. Then District Governor Sealy McCreless of San Antonio came to the rescue. His check for $20,000 sealed the bargain with the federal government. The famous check was framed and hung in the camp administration building. He liked to laugh and ask, "How did you know that check's was good?"

Lions said, with tongue in check, that the ambitious Texas Lions dream became a reality with passage of a bill in Congress and a hot check in Texas. The minute the beautiful site was obtained and the deed was locked in a Kerrville bank vault, another problem arose. The League was straining at the bit to start camp construction and bring in the children. Now they were faced with another formidable question: How would they raise an additional $150,000 or so needed to build the camp?

Did the Lions of Texas have a tiger by the tail?

— Chapter 2 —

"The Traveling Salesmen"

"Little children remain our first and most sacred trust, while crippled children engage our attention and touch our heartstrings."

— *Unknown*

Europe, South America, Antarctica, or wherever Texas Lions met other Lions, the Texans expected one question: "Will you tell us about your crippled children's camp?" E. B. (Tex) Mayer, past director of Lions International, said the camp was the most widely known and most asked about Lions project anywhere in the world.

In the middle Twentieth Century, when Lionism was on the move and Texas Lions were campaigning for funds to build their camp in the Hill Country, the future seemed uncertain. The League, governing body of camp operations, had just raised $100,000 in six months to fulfill their obligations to the federal government and obtain deed to the property. Now they were faced with finding at least an additional $150,000 for construction. The League found friends in many unexpected quarters.

Walt Shaffer, longtime member of the Texas City Lions Club, said that he remembered when a committee set up to plan the fund campaign met at the Rice Hotel in Houston. It adjourned early be-

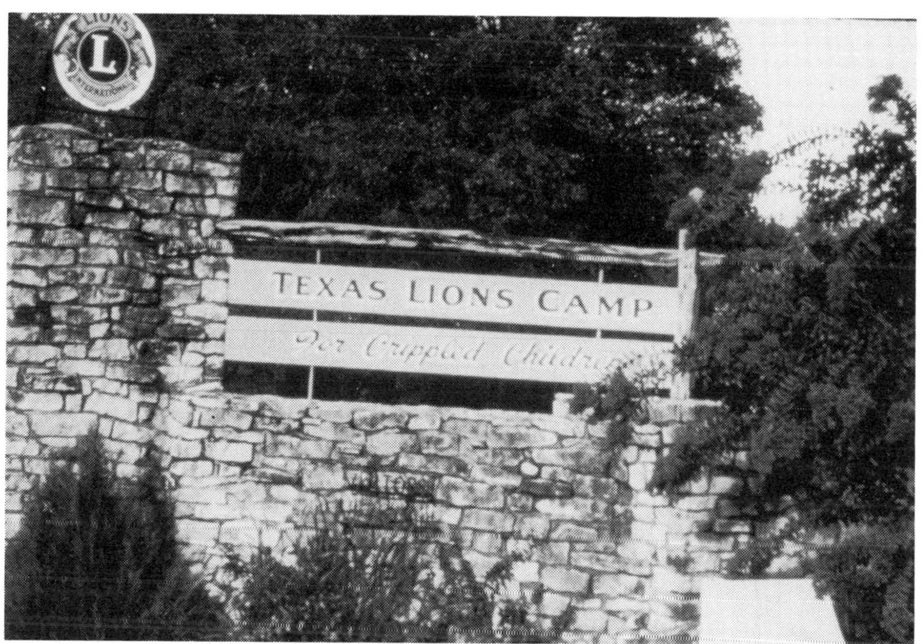

Children left their handicaps at the gate.

cause plans were stymied. Texas City Lions knew that there were some $10,000 leftover from worldwide contributions to that coastal area after the killing tanker explosion in the harbor in 1945. After a couple of years Texas City had reconstructed everything needed, and still had money left over. The Texas City Lions Club persuaded the city to donate the leftovers to help the statewide effort to found a camp for crippled children. Shaffer said he called the committee back and gave them the $10,000.

Another unexpected contribution came in a letter to Jack Wiech, League president, from W. E. (Pete) Driskill, with whom Lion Bill Mickelsen had worked at the Federal Security Agency to gain the property.

Wrote Driskill: "May I express this personal appreciation of your efforts and my congratulations on your success thus far. It is noted that you have more than 35,000 Lions in Texas. It is also noted that you have indicated that $10 would be an active membership in your program. Even though I am not a Lion, attached is my personal check for membership in your project; and if each Lion would contribute that amount, it would raise $350,000, more than enough to complete this project immediately."

With new found friends like that, the League thought their brother Lions could be doing even better. It took three tedious years, during some of which only hardheaded determination and physical stamina kept the League and its dream going.

Again, the League considered employing a professional fund-raiser. In 1952, it hired Kerrville Lion George Brown as field man. He made trips all over the state telling about the program that, "God willing and Lions giving," would soon be available at the camp. He reminded his audiences how hard it was for a child to be crippled, always sitting on the outside and never being an active participant. He was sure his brother Lions did not believe that God put the handicapped here and then denied them the chance to work and play to their limit. Children polio victims were still very much in evidence. The appeal was persuasive; Lions over the state opened their hearts and their wallets again. Money started rolling in faster than ever before. Other Lions who spent personal time and money as volunteer traveling salesmen were Jack Wiech, Jack Roe, Reagan Smith, and Frank Robertson. They were caught up in the steam-rolling project which so effectively represented the Lions Clubs purpose: helping those who could not help themselves. Lion George P. Gentry, a Kerrville automobile agency owner, furnished cars and gasoline to the men who could travel to tell the story.

An exciting and significant day was September 28, 1951, when ground breaking ceremonies were held at the camp site. The Lions and their League already had found many supporters in high places, like Texas Governor Shivers who had helped to kick off a fund drive for the initial $100,000. On this day the popular Texas Secretary of State, John Ben Shepperd, and Past Lions International President Herb Petry were the principal speakers. Lions attended from all over the state. Almost all the officers of each district were there. Spirits were high. The September sun spread its warmth over the green-yellow-red foliage of trees dotting the area and made this particular day seem especially bright. Lions looked with pride over the grounds. The League advanced to the next step in creating their dream when the contract was let for construction of the first buildings on the camp site, two bunkhouses. That night, when Wiech finally crawled into bed, he breathed his first sigh of relief since 1948. Jack Roe's dream had become a reality; the chil-

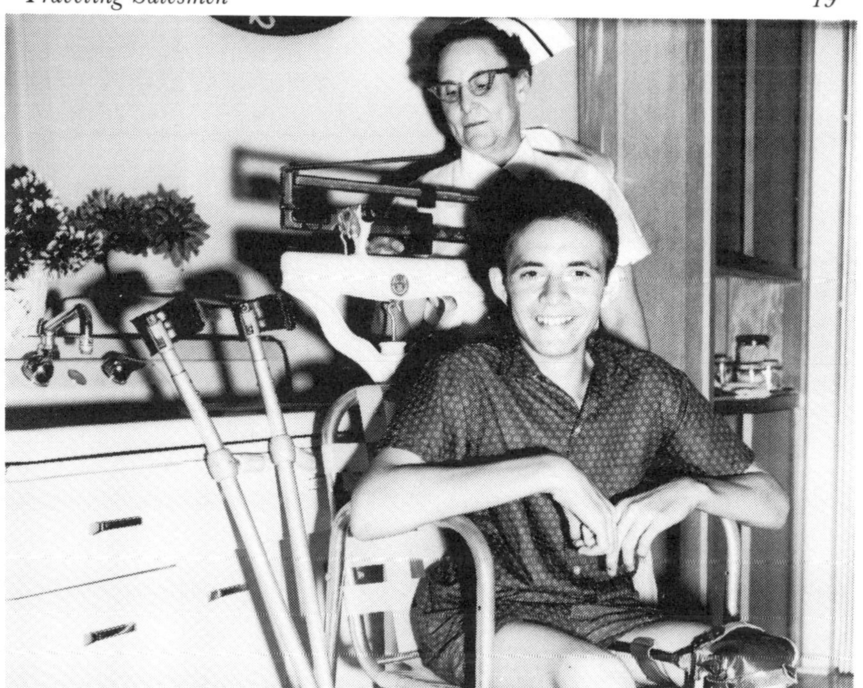

Nurses in the Infirmary made kids feel better, and listened to their secrets.

dren's camp was solidly entrenched; there was no way to go but forward.

Beginning in 1951, League leaders convinced the clubs over Texas that each one should hold a fund-raiser for the camp to inject new life into dwindling camp funds. This remained as an annual event for every Lions club in the state. From wacky womanless weddings to rough-and-tumble rodeos, and from pancake suppers to formal dinner-auctions, the Lions pushed their annual fund-raisers. In 1952 League directors approved the first Christmas card selling project as a camp sponsored money-maker. This enterprise was established in addition to the annual, noise-making benefits held by each club.

With dollars in their pockets, the League built two bunkhouses, a dining room and kitchen, the infirmary, a swimming pool, and portions of an arts and crafts building. It was in 1952 that Wiech retired as president of the League, and Frank Robertson, a well-known San Antonio builder, succeeded him.

The League appointed Mickelsen as camp architect. This Lion had been the tireless legman in Washington during the days of securing the site. With that successfully behind him, Mickelsen spent the next fifteen years planning, designing and supervising all camp construction. He donated much of his time and professional services; and when compensation was necessary, he accepted only a modest fee. Upon his death, the League followed a request in his will: after cremation of his body, the ashes were to be spread over the small hill on which the camp chapel rests and on the largest hill on the camp, Inspiration Point. There have been reports that staffers and campers, who know this story in the Lions camp history, sometimes have felt a strange sensation down near the chapel and up on Inspiration Point. Camp Executive Director Glenn Crawford said that it could be Bill Mickelsen still watching over the camp he loved so much and worked so hard to create. "He probably is smiling happily each summer when his beautiful children come rolling up the hill and past the chapel to camp headquarters," smiled Crawford.

Mickelsen built handsome sturdy structures of steel, concrete and stone. All were designed for safe and easy use. There were no stairs or steps in the camp buildings since the special campers needed easy access. Free flow of air through the bunkhouse quarters was a priority design for Mickelsen. The dining room was built in oval shape, so each child at the respective tables would be about the same distance from the serving area. The pool was triangular shaped, allowing greater shallow water space. A slide "shot" the children from wheelchairs into the water, where their handicaps were washed away. Later another pool was added to the original triangular one because swimming became the most important activity at camp.

While the initial building program was underway during 1951–52, the League's board of directors intensified efforts to tell every Lion in the state about the camp. An Active and Life camp membership program was set up which greatly increased the League's bank account. Date for opening of the camp was set for June 1953. In addition to receiving undesignated donations, the League accepted many earmarked gifts. The Houston Central and Gulf Coast Lions Clubs gave the money for construction of the infirmary; Maurice Pipkin, director of the vocational division of Texas Southmost College in Brownsville, and his two mill cabinet classes, built furniture for the entire camp, including 500 desks, tables, footlockers, kitchen work tables, beds and bunk beds,

TEXAS LIONS CAMP
FOR
CRIPPLED CHILDREN
DONATED BY
CORPUS CHRISTI LIONS CLUB

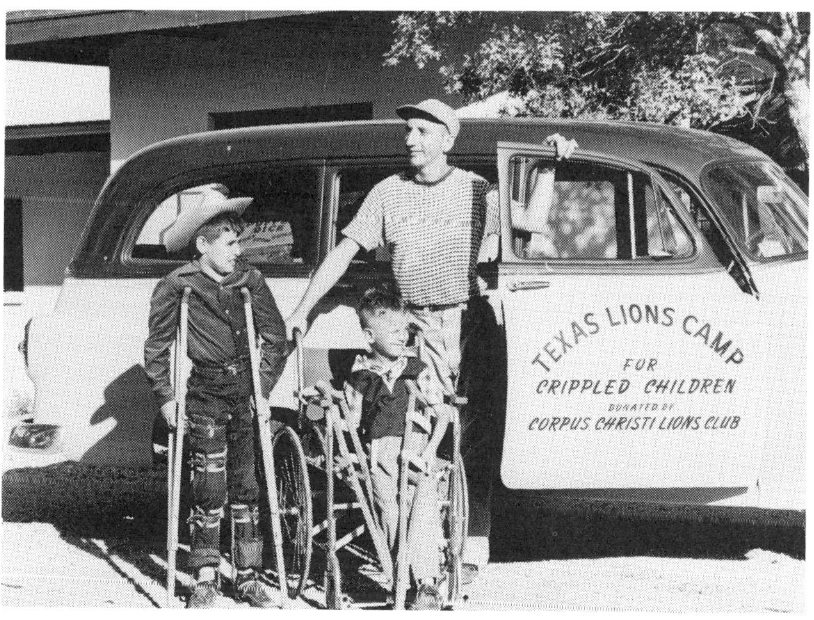

Lions and their clubs donated everything from vehicles to nature displays and cookies.

benches, and picnic tables. Howard Butt of H.E.B stores headquartered in Corpus Christi, hauled all the furniture from Brownsville to the camp.

The spring of 1953 was filled with hectic days and plenty of hardships for the League. No one but Jack Roe, who outlined the original plans for operation of the camp, had ever run a camp before, so it was trial-and-error that first year. Many days the camp staff looked up to see a Lions car slowly driving up the hill with a pickup truck in tow as a donation, or a fat calf to be butchered for food for the children, or a gentle mare to ride, or six dozen pillows for the bunks.

As camp opening drew nearer, Robertson and his staff discovered that Lions over the state had been very busy. Many called daily to ask what was needed. They were determined that their camp would succeed from the very first summer. From their respective communities the Lions secured donations from grocery stores, hardware stores, dairies, cookie-makers, paper suppliers, and pharmaceutical companies, plus many other outlets. Often the Lions themselves brought the supplies to camp. They were anxious to see how their camp was progressing. Many Kerrville individuals and businesses helped. Low bid for the inner, main road was $5,885.00. Hal Peterson and Street Hamilton of Kerrville built it for $2,550.45 because they donated every hour of labor on the all-weather road.

It was almost June, there were many last-minute problems to solve, not the least of which was the resignation of both the program director and the purchasing agent. President Robertson moved from San Antonio to Kerrville and took personal control of the situation. He reorganized the staff and opened camp on schedule. He remained as camp director for the next twenty-three years. He employed Mildred Newman as secretary, who soon became assistant executive director, and remained until her retirement in 1979.

In 1988 there was a counselor for every three children. In 1953 there were eight counselors for the forty children attending the first session. Finding counselors was a hard job. Most of them were college students on vacation who lived in the general area; many were "conscripted' by Lions of the area. In a few years Robertson found that he had waiting lists for counselor positions every year.

On the morning of June 8, 1953, the staff and counselors of the brand new Texas Lions League Camp were up before dawn. Everything was ready for the children, and they nervously awaited the campers. Soon they heard the hum of an automobile down at the entrance to the camp. They knew the car was passing through the native rock entrance, pilasters of which displayed the emblem of the Lions clubs. Four Bible verses were engraved on these pilasters. One said, "Suffer little children to come unto Me, and forbid them not, for of such is the Kingdom of God." The car headed up the hill, rounded all the curves, and finally stopped in the parking lot. A Lions member from a club down on the coast got out of the car. He opened the back door and helped a boy. About nine years old, the boy stood with both legs supported by unwieldy braces. Then the Lion reached in the car for a walker.

Jeremy took it and slowly walked a few steps. He stared at the huge swimming pool; his bright blue eyes, that matched the color of the water, were shining. He had been told he would be taught to swim. Could it really be? He turned his small body from side to side, looking intently over the hills. He had been told also that he would go into the woods to sleep overnight. Jeremy couldn't imag-

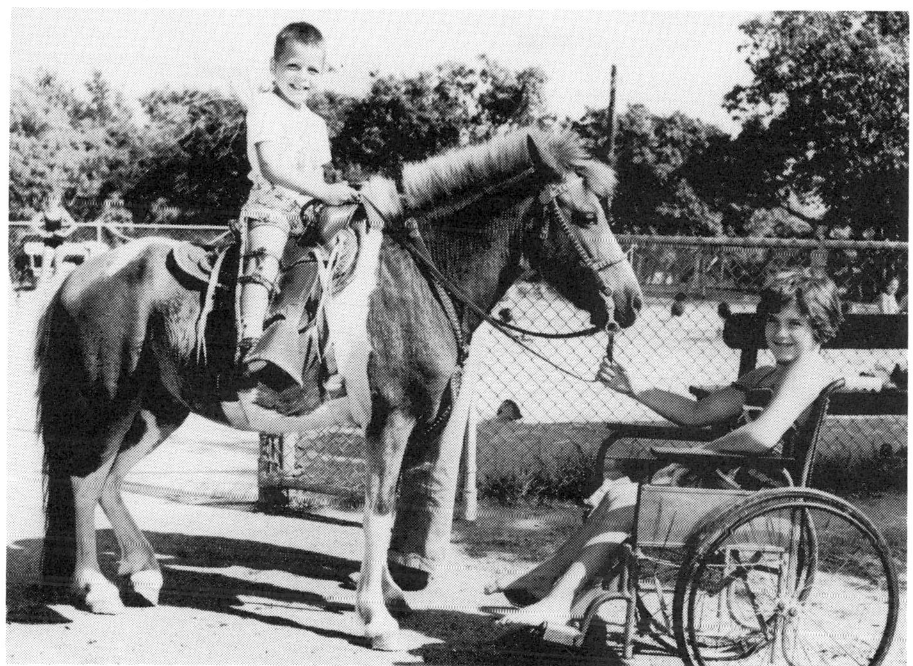

Early "horse wranglers" at Lions camp, pictured with first horse on the camp.

ine that back home, but he wondered if he might be able to do it here at this camp. How would he manage? Two counselors ran to meet him, excited and smiling. He was shy, as usual. Jeremy never knew if people would accept him or not. He looked back at the pool again.

Then he asked softly, "Am I going to get in that pool?"

"Of course," one young man said. "And you'll be swimming in no time at all." Was it possible? again thought Jeremy.

A station wagon rolled to a stop in the camp parking lot. Another Lion, this time from the Panhandle of Texas, opened the vehicle door, then assisted a girl, obviously blind, and a youngster in a wheelchair. The man had driven over 500 miles to bring the two children to camp. A couple was along, too, who were identified as parents of the blind child. Both looked quickly over the camp and the hills, and to the mass of sky above. They frowned and seemed worried.

The little girl was smiling. "Mother," called Lindy, I think I can smell a new, outdoor smell. Are we in the camp hills?"

"Y-y-es," the mother replied, still frowning.

When two more young and laughing counselors welcomed these children, Lindy's mother motioned for one to come to the other side of the automobile and talk. She told the counselor that Lindy was only seven years old and had never spent one night away from home. "She doesn't hardly feed herself. I always help her get dressed. Oh, I don't know if we should leave her. I'm sorry, but I will miss her so, and I will worry."

"Please try not to," said the counselor. "We are going to give each child individual attention, and we will take very good care of Lindy. She will be completely supervised at all times, and we hope Lindy will have lots of fun and do new things." Was it possible the mother asked herself. Was it possible for a blind seven-year-old to live two weeks outdoors in a camp by herself? Lindy, with long curls waving around her shoulders, was already holding the hand of the other counselor and heading for the pool. Lindy thought: "Am I really at a camp, in the hills, very near to the sky?"

Texas Lions League camp was open!

Soon the League would have the answers to questions asked by many: How could you unite the Lions of Texas to support a project not located in their district? How could you find forty children to attend the proposed camp? Would the parents let their handicapped children stay away from home for a two-week session? How would the children feel among strangers?

Jeremy, Lindy, and the thirty-eight other children who camped with the Lions in the first session of that first summer had many surprises. Yes, it was going to be possible for them to learn to swim, ride horses, and sleep under the stars where they felt they were almost to heaven.

Who's handicapped?

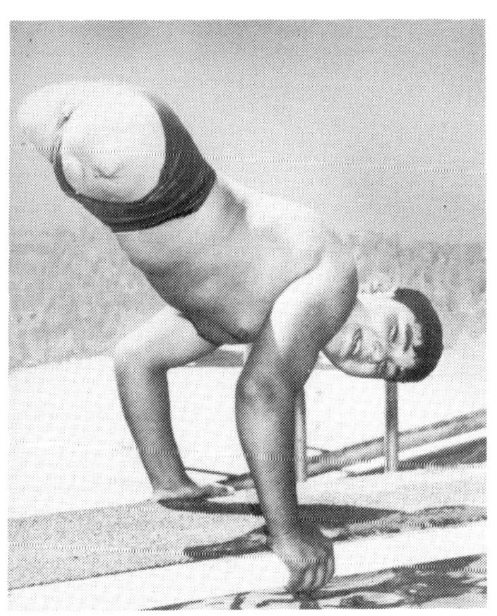

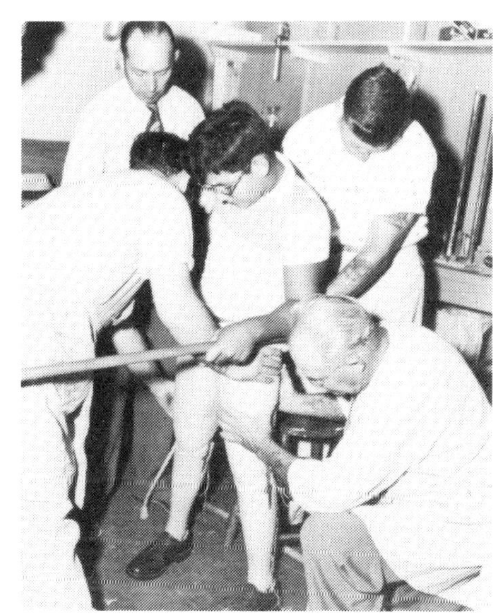

NOT ME!

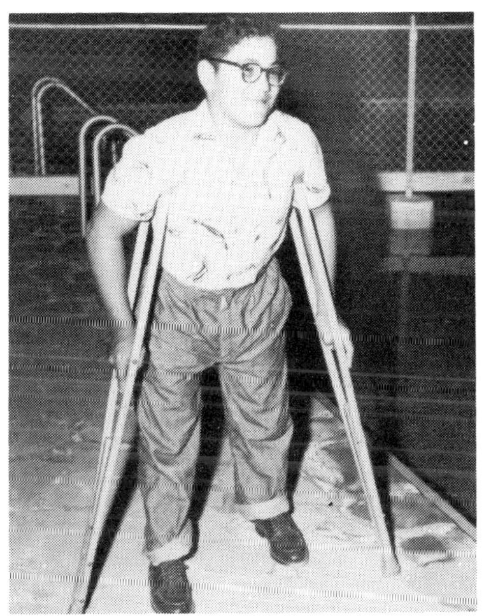

— Chapter 3 —

"That First Summer"

"They learned they don't always have to receive help. They can give it, too."

— *Glenn Crawford, Camp Executive Director*

Crippled children cannot be put with blind children at a camp, said psychologists and child education specialists. They do not play and work well together. Members of the Lions camp governing board, the League, discussed the situation and decided that concept was ridiculous.

Almost any hour during the summer camp for the handicapped, visitors could see a blind child pushing a wheelchair occupied by a child with sight who gave the directions. There may be another blind child or perhaps a mute tagging along. Sometimes several chairs and their pushers, many in braces, formed a train. It was at these times that persons walking the paths needed to watch carefully; those trains were fast and nonstop until they reached their destination. A sign on one wheelchair said "Caution, Wild Driver." Visitors were instructed to watch out for the skateboards. There were numerous children at the Lions camp through the decades whose legs were missing so far up that they could not be fit-

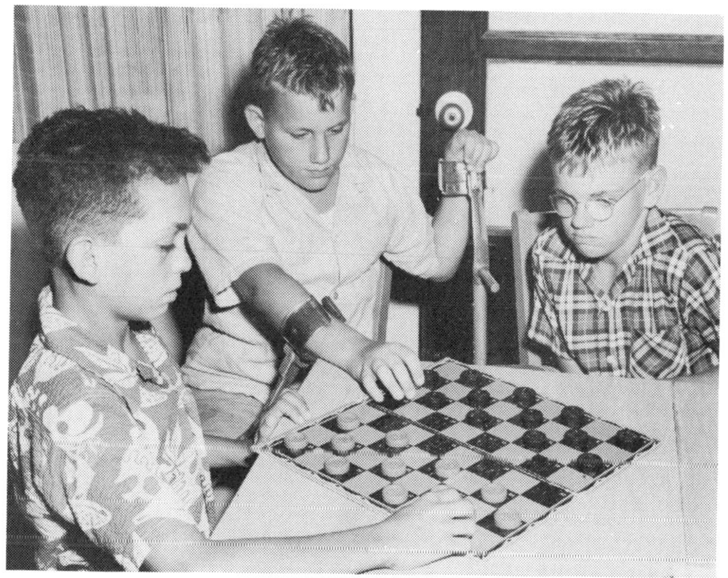

Newly made friends at Lions camp played a game of checkers.

ted for artificial limbs. These were the campers who whirled around the walks and paths on the hot-rod skateboards. They always beat everybody to the chow line.

When the Lions camp reached the big "40" in age in 1989, it had proved the professionals wrong. Not any time during the years had the camp had a single minute of worry or controversy regarding the togetherness of the blind, mute, deaf, and crippled children. Experience soon proved that the Lions were right. Their campers displayed a commendable spirit of togetherness. The common bond seemed to bring a real understanding between the boys and girls, and they *did* camp successfully with each other.

Lions who helped transport the children to camp that first summer went back to tell the other owners of the camp that it was exceeding expectations. Lions over the state could not wait to see their dream in action; many visits were made to the hilltop in the summer of 1953. Robertson was the full time director.

Although it was a long way from Brownsville to Kerrville, Wiech went often to help make decisions, and he spent many hours in telephone conversations. Calls came into the camp daily from

Lions over the state, asking how things were progressing and how they could help. Two big problems were menus and wheelchairs. Parents forgot to explain on the application forms that their children needed special diets; many children came to camp with crutches only. When hiking the trails, most of these children needed wheelchairs because it was too tiring to walk with crutches. Even children with leg braces often needed to ride the long distances. Lion leaders and directors of the League responded to the call for wheelchairs. Enough of the right kind of equipment was a problem throughout the summer, but the staff kept lists and records so that by the next year, this was not a major concern.

It was a first experiment in the world of camping. In spite of problems and trial-and-error programs, everyone was optimistic; the *I can* spirit prevailed; and only positive attitudes were allowed. This atmosphere remained throughout the camp's history.

In midsummer the news media of Texas were invited for a day's tour as guests of the League. Newspaper, radio, and television personnel came, saw and went back to tell their readers and viewers. From the beginning of the idea for the camp the media of the state played an important part. Communications was a keyword for the statewide project, and the Lions of Texas always had the cooperation of the media which, like other donors, believed in the innovative facility. The "press" of Texas wanted it to work, and they were proud of its continuous prestige in the world. The media recognized colorful and interesting copy in the crippled children's camp.

The following excerpts are from the August 5, 1953, issue of the *Waco News-Tribune*, and were written by Betty Dollins.

> Texas Lions, probably your grocer, banker or doctor, and the cool, green hills of West Texas are stealing the hearts of Texas' crippled kids. The Lions are having wonderful returns on their quarter-million-dollar investment at the Texas Lions Camp for Crippled Children at Kerrville. You have to see it for yourself. You have to see kids on crutches pushing their young wheelchair-bound playmates around the camp, a young teen-age boy learning to swim with only one leg, a blond pigtailed girl completely blind and paralyzed in both legs weaving a straw hat in the big craft shop, a swimming instructor whose crutches and braces are lying along the edge of the pool.
>
> Dean came to the pool at swim time in a wheelchair. He wore a bright blue bathing suit, and the biggest smile in camp. A

> blond-headed young girl, Joan Kester of Trinity University, lifted him gently from the wheelchair, and dipped the shrunken pale legs into the water. She helped Dean float on his back and blow bubbles in the water. Another instructor nearby helped a tall teen-age boy, Gene Reichle of Sweetwater, with some diving ring work. Gene had been severely burned and lost his right leg. Some of the youngsters bring to camp along with their crutches more self pity than is good for them. But there just isn't room for it. They see other children with handicaps perhaps worse than their own. Sixteen-year-old James Geiger of LaCoste is a junior instructor in swimming. When Monday's swim was over, he was out of the pool and on his crutches in no time. He was busy in a few minutes pushing fourteen-year-old Wilbert Woodard's wheelchair back to the bunkhouse. Wilbert was crippled by polio.

Water play and swimming, which were held twice a day in the camp's first year, had always headed the list of favorites at the Lions camp. In addition to swimming that first summer, counselors taught arts and crafts, nature crafts, field games, archery, and games of their own creation. Tournaments were held in checkers, darts, dominoes, golf, shuffleboard, table tennis, horseshoes, and ring toss. That year, and each succeeding summer, the ever-popular pajama parade was held. Camp outs ran close seconds to swimming, because it was new for most of the kids. A road had already been carved around the highest hill to the top which was called Inspiration Point. Here was the most exciting place to sleep out and experience all the wonders of living in the outdoors: building a campfire, cooking supper, singing songs, telling ghost stories, and finally getting to sleep under the stars. There were cookouts and sunrise breakfasts on other parts of the acreage, too. This was the only camp in Texas where a crippled, blind, deaf, or mute child could go. Here he met others like himself; here he learned to help instead of being helped. No one stared at him because he was crippled. No one pitied him or laughed at him because he couldn't talk well or because he stumbled. Here in his own world he found a place for himself and became a more confident person. The goal of League officials and camp staffers was to have, hopefully, all the children develop a skill or a new hobby; and, more importantly, could go back to that first world with faith that they could become productive adult citizens.

On the staff with Executive Director Frank Robertson were Jacqueline Gleckler of Houston, assistant director, Earl Stobaugh

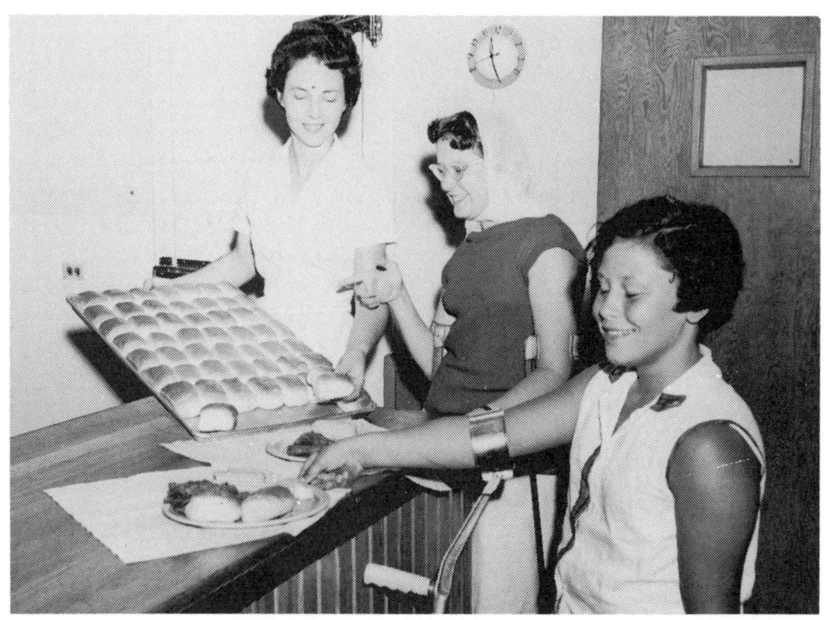

The camp provided good food, and plenty of it to fill appetites perked up by outdoor recreation.

of Fredericksburg, program director; Earline Sample of Kerrville, registered nurse; Joan Kester of San Antonio, waterfront director; Marilyn Itz of Albert, assistant waterfront director; Elizabeth Carter of Neches, arts and crafts director; Marilyn Soboslay of Fort Worth, arts and crafts assistance; Marie Mahon and Sue Scott of Kerrville, girls unit leaders; Dick Stone, boys unit leader; Shirley Creswell of Port Arthur and Jane Martinez of San Marcos, assistant girl unit leaders; Jerry Zimmermann of San Antonio and Tyrus Hawkins of Kerrville, assistant boy unit leaders; Theo Ann Kennedy of Kerrville, Barbara Shaw of Houston,Joy Green of Marble Falls, and Linn Roe of Kerrville, all counselors-in-training; Anna Moss of Kerrville, food director, assisted by Fanny Warren and Buda Warren of Kerrville; J. C. Murray of Kerrville, caretaker; Houriah Brown of Kerrville, handyman; Louis Hays of Kerrville, camp secretary.

Before camp opened Jack Roe had written a manual for counselors at the camp, explaining the objectives, aims, policies, and regulations, and suggesting guidelines for care of campers. He made a list of what counselors might expect physically and emotionally from children of various age levels then added desirable qualities in a counselor. Roe even suggested menus and camp activities. He also was responsible for hiring Gleckler on the staff. She had been working on a master's degree in camping for the handicapped child and had taught crippled children to swim at Houston.

It was not known who composed the Lions camp song, which is sung to the tune of Auld Lang Syne, but it originated that first summer and remained as the official camp song. The daily schedule for 1953 was somewhat like the schedule for the next several decades, beginning with reveille at 7 A.M., followed by breakfast, cabin cleanup, assembly and singsong, cabin programs and crafts, swimming, lunch, camp store, rest hour, afternoon projects, swimming, supper, evening program of special entertainment, and taps.

A camp newspaper entitled *The Crutch* was produced after each two-week session and mentioned every child at camp. It was rumored that a funny little ghost named Lione was editor of the newspaper. Lione said, in print, that it was her diary, but the campers helped her write it. "You never saw me around, but I was there. I saw you in cabin cleanup and you didn't always sweep underneath the beds. Oh, I was there when you burned the bacon on Inspiration Point. I am the spirit of the Lions Camp." A twelve-year-old camper named Shirley was artist for the first newspaper. Printed in one issue late in the summer was a letter from Roberto Duchene.

He wrote, "I want to thank everyone especially Mr. Robertson, Mac, Mr. Vaughn, and Doc for getting me the artificial legs. Jerry has been helping me do my daily exercises. I sure get lots of hope when I know everybody is backing me up." Roberto came for the first two-week session, but because he was being fitted with legs and taught how to use them, he stayed most of the summer.

Jokes were printed in those first issues of *The Crutch,* which in a few summers was changed to The Lions Tale. "An apple and banana went on top of the Empire State Building. The apple jumped off. Why didn't the banana jump? Answer: the banana was yellow." Sometimes campers wrote about what they had learned at camp. Dennis said "I never could button my shirt, but I tried and I did it for the first time. Bobby kept helping me and I finally did it." Eight-year-old Vicky learned to get into her wheelchair all by herself; it took a lot of huffing and puffing. Dennis wrote in the little newspaper that after Awards Night and the last campfire, "we

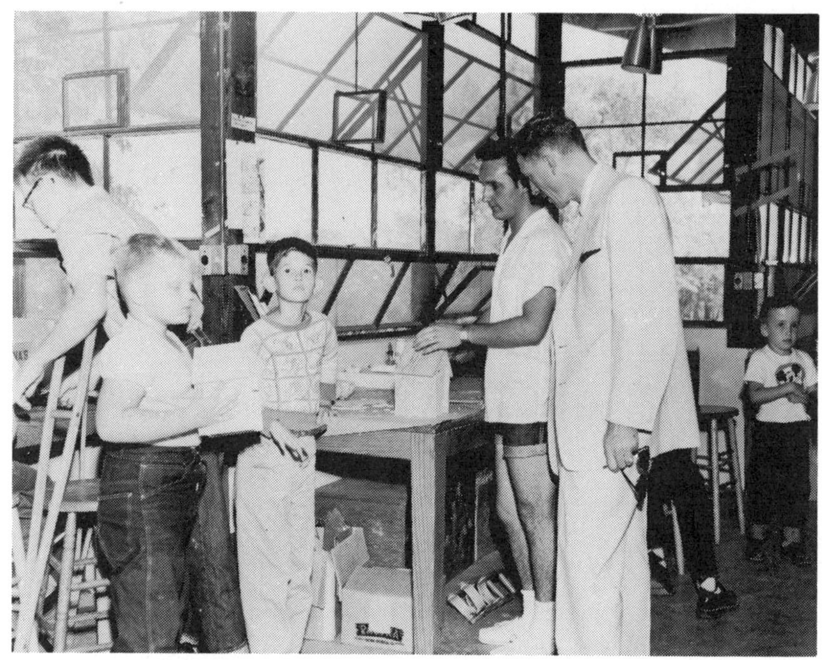

Arts and Crafts was always popular with the children.

didn't want to go, but other campers must have a chance at fun, too."

Nancy Suzanne learned to float on her back. She had not walked in six years, but called herself a "crawfish walking in the water." Freda had always fallen a lot as she was awkward on her braces, but she laughed every time. Counselors and friends worked with her and she learned how to make her falls easier. "Now I fall good," she said and still laughed. Windell Dickerson and Dan Jones came as campers, but remained as counselors-in- training. A very popular guy one session was Bobby Stovenour, whose half-sister was the film actress, June Havor. Bobby promised to get her autographed picture for everyone in camp. Swimming awards included the Tadpole Award for beginners, the Frog Award for the mid-group, and the Fish Award for advanced swimmers. Ones who progressed the most received Porpoise Awards, and the first recipient was Darlene, a leg amputee. She was terrified of the water, but was determined to try. The kindness and expertise which the counselors used to help conquer fear also helped her to achieve some degree of skill in the water.

Special events for the summer of 1953 were a water show produced by the counselors, including clown act; a trip by bus to nearby Kerrville to see a rodeo; a visit by the Fort Worth Lions Club who came to dedicate their gift to the camp, Bunkhouse I.

The little ghost, Lione, who was always pictured in the newspaper wrapped in a white sheet, wrote in the last issue published that first summer: "As it came time for you to leave, I saw the reluctance in your eyes and upon your quivering lips. You never saw me, but on these occasions I had to use my sheet to wipe the tears from my eyes."

Texas Lions Camp was officially dedicated on July 3. The ceremony's participants included Lion members, campers, staff, and special guests Wiech, Congressman O. C. Fisher, and International Lions Clubs Past President Petry. Camp Director Frank Robertson introduced League officers, after which President Wiech made brief remarks. Master of ceremonies was Lion C. N. Hielscher who introduced Congressman Fisher and Petry. The invocation was given by District Governor Jack B. Wright of San Antonio. Jackie Gleckler, program director, reported on the camp activities, and Lion J. L. Crockett sang two patriotic songs. A camper, Diego Gallegos, led the Pledge of Allegiance, and a Jewish rabbi, a Catholic priest, and a protestant minister offered prayers.

At the end of the first two weeks, forty happy children won awards at the concluding ceremony; at the end of the summer 236 children, with handicaps of all kinds, had experienced a thrill of a lifetime. The Lions of Texas had answered four questions which had come up before the camp was constructed. Yes, the Lions of Texas *could* unite to support a project not in their district; yes, parents *would* let their handicapped children stay away from home for a two-week session; yes, the Lions could find enough children to fill each session; and, no, children would not feel they were huddled together with strangers, for they relaxed and accepted each other as friends and buddies.

The Lions camp children were always called "just kids." During the first summer of operation, the governing League found that their campers were, after all, just kids, like any other kid camping. Most of them didn't want to go to sleep at night and hated rest periods; they ate like little horses and gained weight; they were mischievous and loved pranks. The most asked question was "when are we going swimming" and an overworked phrase was "I double dare you."

The Lions Camp founders, leaders and members patted themselves on the back. They did it! They established the first successful camp for handicapped children in Texas, which was to continue on a steady, progressive basis, and become recognized the world over. It was the first and only camp to be accredited as a private school by the Texas Education Agency; first and only camp in the world to produce an extensive curriculum manual; first Lions camp in the world to introduce therapeutic horseback riding; only camp in the world to have a scientifically and professionally made telescope. The *can do* spirit of the unique camp was to endure; and the *think big* philosophy of the Texas Lions clubs was to persist. Jack Roe, originator of the idea for the camp, said, "All life expands at contact with the outdoors experience. We breathe deeper, we eat more, we feel better." This happened to Michael, who was blind. When his parents asked him how he liked camp, he smiled, "It makes you feel like you are part of the world."

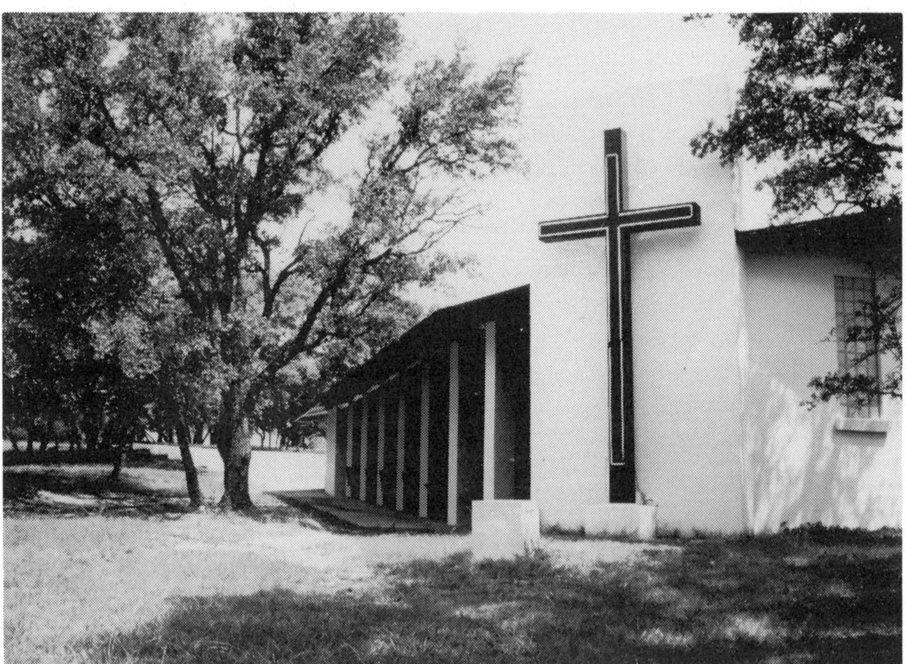

Cross on the outdoor chapel could be seen for miles.

— Chapter 4 —

"Boundless Imagination and Twenty-Four Hour Duty"

"Should I wear my leg this morning?"
— *A camper*

Community living at its best was found on a hilltop in the middle of Texas, where boys and girls came from all over the Lone Star State to camp together. They had a common bond: each one had a physical disability. Some were vision and hearing impaired children; others suffered bone diseases or had cerebral palsy; and many had missing limbs.

"There are no crippled children here," said program director Rand Southard. "We take these little kids and give them a new image. We strive to offset the mental block that most handicapped kids themselves have formed in their own minds. Handicapped children are an extension of society. If the children have these feelings, what must society also think? Our overall goal is to teach our world that a child with a physical disability has the same needs, desires, and feelings as any other child. We teach the child and the world at the same time."

Southard was both a former camper and counselor at this unique facility, and he knew from firsthand experience that "Here

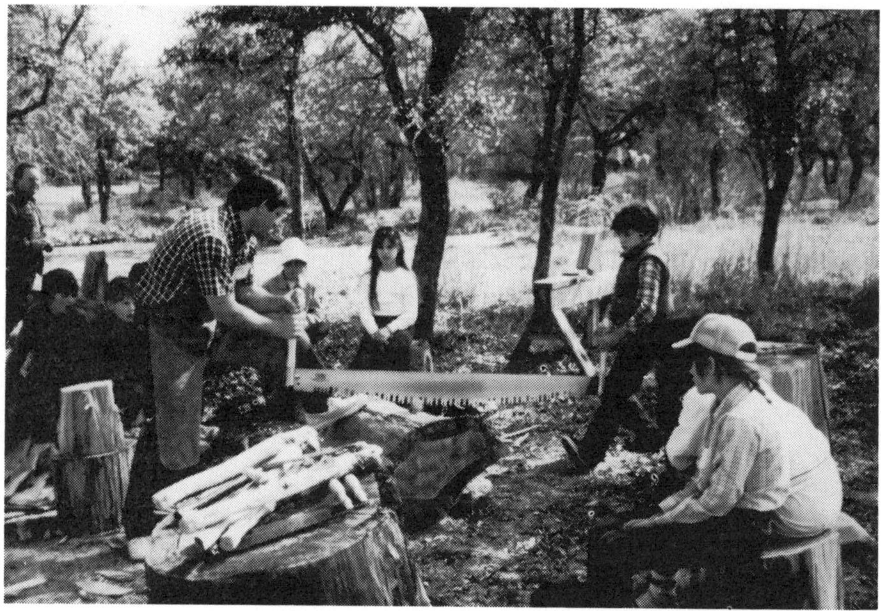

Rand Southard, camp program director, showed kids how to make shingles.

is where these children can lick their problems. They are fighting to be just normal kids. They deserve to be kids, no different from any other kid. They just want to be accepted."

Glenn Crawford, executive director of the camp in 1989, addressed the subject of terminology for the youngsters. "Yesterday we called them crippled, and today we call them handicapped. Tomorrow there will be a new word, because with the years there are always changes. Perhaps tomorrow we will call our campers 'children'."

In 1949 the newly formed Lions League insisted that, if they could help it, no child would be deprived of the adventures of camping just because of a physical impairment. They worked hard to accomplish this. In the camp's fortieth year, 1989, one counselor said, "If the Lions over the state just realized what they are doing and could see the miracles of restoration that we see every day, they would be surprised, and very pleased."

Lions clubs from over the world, and other groups interested in operation of camps for the handicapped, have visited the Texas Lions camp since it opened in 1953 to study, ask questions, take notes and go home with guidelines for establishing a similar facility. Among these visitors were Lions from Sweden, Australia, Panama, Japan and Canada. The Texas camp was the role model, and was the largest such camp in the world, with the most extensive program for handicapped children over 250 activities. As the first known founded Lions camp in the world, the Texas group was active in the Conference of Lions Camps of the United States, which included twenty other similar facilities. The Conference met for a week once a year and exchanged information on such subjects as program design, site facility development, fund-raising, legal considerations, insurance, budgets, long-range planning, public relations, foundation board structures, food service, staff, personnel evaluations, utilization of camp year around, maintenance, and camper and program evaluations.

Handicapped children, like non-handicapped children, are curious, adventuresome human beings. "They want to be someone to themselves and others within their life-space," said a Lion, "so they set up their camp as the vehicle to help these special children to meet their human and individual needs." At this camp the kids were provided with the opportunity to learn, grow, succeed and find pleasure in a planned, controlled setting.

The program for the summer sessions for handicapped children was tailor-made to develop the campers' talents, to stretch the imaginations and unused muscles, and to help the boys and girls forget cumbersome handicaps. The biggest myth, explained Southard, was that kids came here just for fun. The carefully planned and executed program was designed to accomplish many things: first, to help a child find something he liked to do, develop it, and instill a desire to carry it into a lifetime of happy activity; and, second, to expose the child to activities which he had never done, like horseback riding, overnight camping, and making up a bunk bed.

Benefits they derived were primarily for themselves, but also benefitting from the campers new selves were their parents, siblings, teachers, and friends. One thing most campers conquered at the Lions facility was the over-protectiveness of parents. They learned self-care skills, self-confidence, improved self-awareness, and unrealized potentials. They went home after two weeks of new adventures, which gave them an opportunity to test their personal, social, and emotional strengths in previously unknown, but supportive situations. They learned how to get along with others in a communal setting and acquired knowledge which could be used to gain success at school. They learned to apply new skills to certain environments and came to realize that one must engage in some personally undesirable tasks in order to participate in group activities. The handicapped children learned that it was all right to have emotions but also learned methods of self-control through discussions with peers having the same problems. Their physical stamina was improved and motor skills were increased through remedial and recreational activities in a well-planned cycle of work, play, and rest.

Although almost every minute of the camper's day was planned, the program and its activators, the highly trained counselors, were flexible enough to give time and attention to the individual needs of their special children. Some required longer to accomplish an activity, and some found they needed to move on to something else that they could handle easier. Most found that they could do many things they thought impossible. The program was based on wholesome self-help.

Southard, who had been program director for three years in 1989, was a former teacher of special education and had worked with all types of handicapped children. He was a professional instructor of swimming, archery, riflery, American Red Cross water safety, and had been named a certified camp director by the American Camping Association. He held a masters degree in education, and was in charge of all summer camp and the outdoor education programs at the Lions camp.

Lions Camp guidelines for developing a positive camp program included targeting the group or individuals to be served, looking at abilities rather than disabilities, finding places in a camp program where the child could fit without accommodations, considering peripheral activities which required few accommodations, and planning new activities for groups. Crippled campers achieved more success if access to necessary items were available. For instance, it would be difficult to enjoy nature from a wheelchair if the path were so rugged that more attention was paid to navigation than to nature. Paths and campsites at the Lions facility were level and always clean and free from obstructions which would hinder mobility of both blind and orthopedically handicapped children.

Programs were planned almost to the minute at the camp, but planners also felt it was important to consider dominating handicaps. Deaf children would not enjoy oral presentations nor blind children visual. Orthopedically handicapped children were made

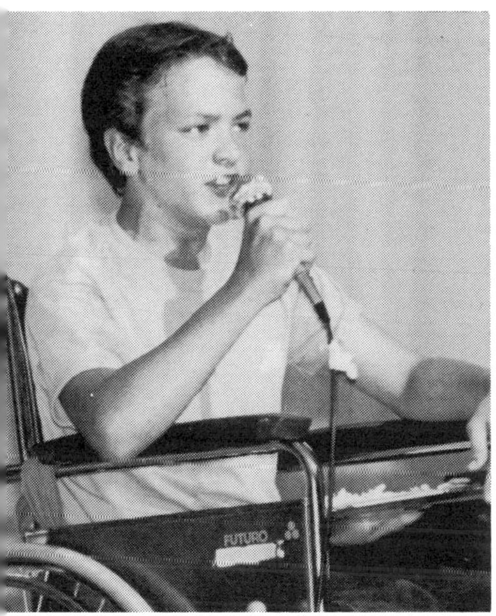

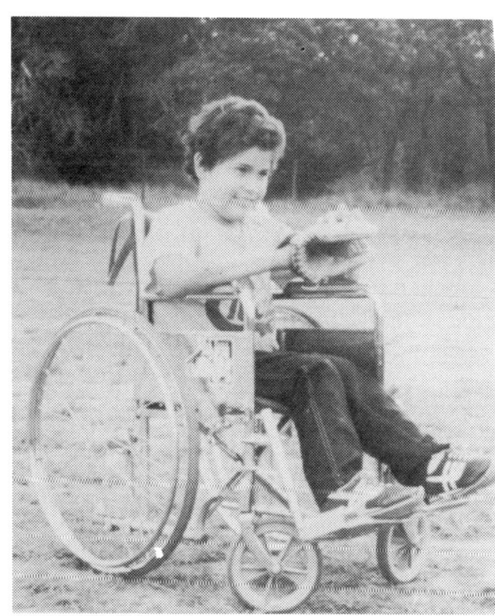

Camper at left was master of ceremonies for a stunt night. Camper at right said "batter up."

as comfortable as possible at all activities and could participate in most. Diabetic children required special diets. Other handicaps were under constant consideration by leaders of the various activities. These things were done without making the camper feel different, and with an effort for the camper to participate willingly. Permanent program department staffers at the Lions camp kept paperwork going at all times because they had found that records were important for reference, future planning, and historical purposes.

They set up the family tree for the summer camp. Each of the nineteen wings in the eight bunkhouses had a wing leader and counselors who lived with the children. There were thirteen camper beds per wing. Sometimes there were counselors-in-training and perhaps activity counselors who also lived there. The wing leader and counselors were responsible to a cluster leader who served as liaison for all of camp life. Cluster leaders were responsible to a camp life coordinator; and activity instructors were responsible to an activity coordinator. On the same level of authority as the coordinators were counselors in charge of transportation and special activities and an assistant program supervisor. These were core staffers, responsible to the program supervisor. On line with this supervisor were the outdoor education supervisor and the horsemanship director. Every staffer mentioned, of course, was under the direction of the program director, who was responsible to the executive director of the camp.

With each year of the Lions camp came changes and innovations in the program. The logistics in operating the largest camp in the world for handicapped children was overwhelming. When a parent asked the program staff what they did in off-season, they answered, "There are no off-seasons." The camp program supervisor worked nine months to put together the three-month summer camping program. Beginning after camp ended, the supervisor received and evaluated counselor applications, set goals for the year, updated the staff manual, formed a check list for supplies for the entire three months, spent several months recruiting and interviewing new counselors from colleges and universities, kept in contact with counselors-in-training, worked on budgets and daily activity schedules for the summer, planned menus with the food service manager, supervised repairs of equipment, and hired counselors and held pre-camp training courses for them.

High on the list of musts for summer was hiring adequate, skilled medical personnel for the infirmary and stocking the infirmary with necessary supplies. In no way was the Texas Lions Camp a medical or correctional facility, although most of its children took medications. It was set up for education and recreation for handicapped children under a system very similar to that of other summer camps. Two of the most important things the Lions children, aged seven to sixteen, learned were how to live happily together and how to compete with others who were their peers.

As summer approached each year, the camp supervisor made last minute checks of the program, planned special events, collected and assigned equipment to staffers, worked up a complete schedule for each of the 120 or more counselors, supervised spraying for insects, set up detailed check-in programs, assigned campers to units, and prepared for an onslaught of many and varied emergencies that were bound to come.

At the Lions camp the maximum use of the outdoors was an unwritten rule. Even structured classes, such as sign language, the challenge course, dramatics, and physical conditioning were held on the grass, if possible. Swimming was the most popular activity for campers, and over half of the kids went home after their two-week session with a swimming medal. Next to swimming was horseback riding, with arts and crafts as third runner-up. First lesson taught in any activity were safety rules.

Campers did not take every class available at the camp. There was not enough time in two weeks. At check-in time campers were asked their preferences, after which counselors discussed them, then the counselors and campers decided together which activities would best meet the campers needs and desires.

Swimming was water therapy at its best. That was why the Lions camp had two big pools, one in triangular shape so that there was plenty of room at the shallow end. Most of the time counselors worked one-on-one in the water with a camper. They were gentle and patient so that the child would not fear the water. When the children came to the waterfront area, it was off with braces, down with crutches, out of wheelchairs, and into the cool buoyancy of the water. This was a first for many, and possibly one that a child had been wanting for a long time. It was not uncommon to hear often: "I can walk in the water!"

Program Director Southard remembers when he was a camper at the Lions facility. A leg amputee, he entered a swimming race in which participants had to swim one length of the pool with their shoes and clothes on, jump out of the water, strip to their swim trunks, then swim another length. Without two shoes and two socks to shed, Southard had an advantage and came in first. He said he realized for the first time that a disability can serve in a person's favor sometimes. The other contestants yelled "unfair," but Southard felt he won square and fair.

Most children, handicapped and non-handicapped, think horses would be very exciting. They might have played cowboys or Indians, in which they envisioned riding like the wind. Horseback riding was a fun experience at the Lions camp, but it was also therapeutic. This type of horseback riding in 1989 was a new trend over the nation, serving as a vehicle in working with handicapped individuals. The horse supervisor at the Lions camp had received extensive training in this area of rehabilitation. As with every major sport, safety rules around horses was the first thing taught to all campers; then the children learned how to feed and care for the animals. Soon came the big experience: kids got into the saddle where they learned riding skills, games on horses, and rodeo tricks. Some

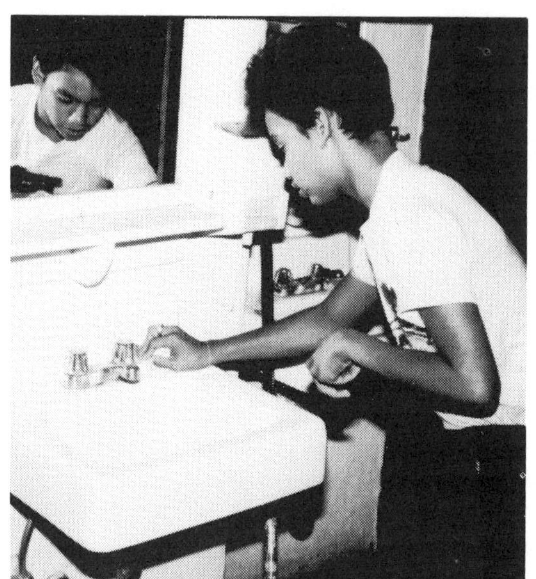

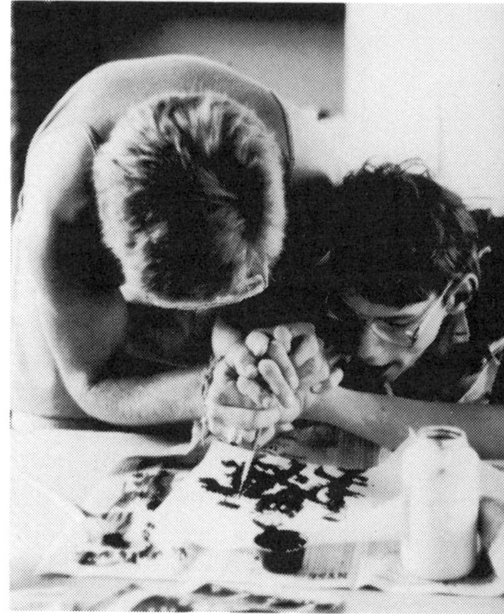

Left: "We never had to clean up at home." Right: Counselors had inexhaustible patience. This one guided shaky fingers to help camper produce something beautiful for his brother.

summers rodeos were held for each session; every summer there were competitive games on horses.

Arts and crafts activities were popular because it gave campers something in hand to show family and friends what they learned to do by themselves. Among the skills taught in this area were working with leather, junk objects campers found, paints, jewelry, wood, clay, macrame, and ceramics. They also learned basket-weaving and rug-plaiting. Campers themselves sometimes created table games and musical instruments for their enjoyment. The program was designed to allow the camper an opportunity to make as many items as he was able to make during the session. Arts and crafts counselors tried to make all classes fun, striving for a relaxed atmosphere in which a boy or girl could find his or her own creative outlet. This activity served as a finely honed therapy for motor coordination.

Nature crafts had unlimited possibilities. Campers were encouraged to experiment in the woods while on supervised hikes and camp outs; and they studied in nature crafts classes all about bugs, birds, tracks, Indian lore, bread-making, habitats for wild animals, farm animals, astronomy, hide-tanning, aquarium construction, survival in the woods, butterflies, weather, fossils, fishing, leaves and trees, rope-making, carving and whittling, star gazing, game laws, water conservation, geography, environment, and use of tools for outdoor living. Here, too, the activities stressed involvement by every camper.

Included in recreation and athletics classes were team sports such as soccer, football, baseball, basketball, volleyball, and "wacky games" created by campers or counselors, sometimes on a moment's thought. Other sports included tennis, track and field, tumbling, riflery, archery, dancing, and miniature golf. Aquatics programs covered the basic activities of adapted aquatics, beginning and intermediate swimming, advanced swimming, recreational swimming, and basic canoeing. In advanced aquatics there were classes in snorkeling, life saving, competitive swimming, water ballet, and overnight canoe trips. All campers took part in some of the swimming activities.

Many of the Lions camp children had never had the opportunity of performing on a stage or speaking before an audience. This type of performance was encouraged at camp, but many boys and girls needed help in summoning the courage. Counselors in the fine arts department were in charge of creating a spirit of enthusiasm in the campers to participate in the "upfront" activity comfortably. On arrival at one session, a boy who had a missing arm would retreat to a corner in embarrassment. Then he looked around and noted that no one paid any attention to his handicap, and most had more problems than he. Soon he came out of his corner, and by the end of the two weeks, he was a skilled archer and served as master of ceremonies at a stunt night program. Just two weeks in the Lions camp environment gave him the courage he needed and brought out his innate desires to achieve. He said, "It's not hard to do when I am among all these friends who are just like me."

Overnight camping was one of the highlights of a camper's two weeks. This event required extra planning by the cluster leaders and the wing counselors. They assigned every camper a job. Some were put on the cleanup detail; others gathered wood for the fire, while some made the fire, helped with the cooking or preparation of food, planned games, or participated in conservation projects. Overnights were planned so that there was a happy balance between structured activities and free time. Living in the woods was conducive to communing with nature and exploring wildlife. Some of the excitement for campers was discovery of these wonders by themselves at their own pace and in their own way. Because of this, a nature craft counselor worked with the leaders in planning the camp outs. Besides cots and bedding, leaders were responsible for transporting all equipment for meals, first aid, inner-camp radios, and, of course, the campers. Most rode to the camp out site in vans. If something was forgotten, it stayed that way; no trips were taken back to the main camp for these items. This was a lesson in survival at times, when camp out participants had to simply tough it out. Sometimes these made the fondest memories. Overnight camp outs were held on the highest hill, called Inspiration Point, or at a wooded campsite, Suddenly.

Evening programs were very special to everyone at camp. Every night was a fun night, and many times it was planned to be a surprise. Some of the events included competitive stunt nights; entertainment programs by the campers, counselors, or outside talents; watermelon or ice cream parties; games, dances, or video shows in the recreation hall. Regardless of the night's entertainment, a day at the Lions camp ended with a campfire, usually held individually by bunkhouses or by one wing of a bunkhouse. Conclusion of a day of fun and learning, came with the Friendship Circle. Campers, leaders, and any visitors present formed a circle, crossing right hands over left to clasp the hand of the next person. It was necessary for some to stoop to hold the hands of the smallest in a wheelchair or help brace a camper leaning on crutches. The song that was always sung was "Green Trees."

Green trees around us;
blue skies above;
friends all about us
in a world filled with love.
Taps sounding softly;
hearts beating true;
as campers say good night to you.

Afterwards, there might be prayers in the wings from little persons on their bunks, while the traditional bugle blew the last good night "taps."

In addition to the structured classes, there were many traditions observed at the Lions camp — flag raising and lowering, bunkhouse cleanups, and Sunday church services in the Wright Memorial Chapel on the campgrounds. The special chapel was de-

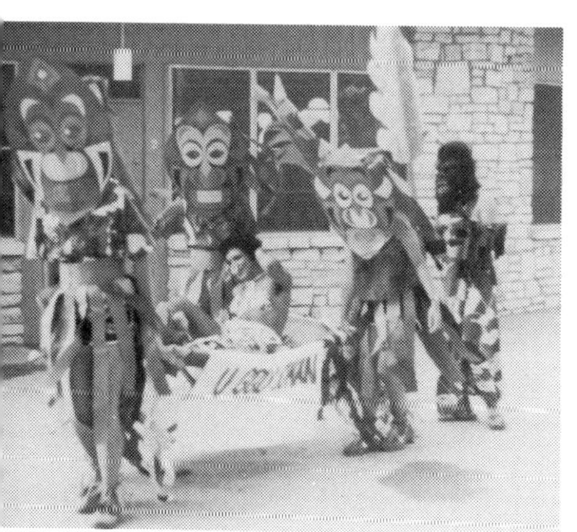

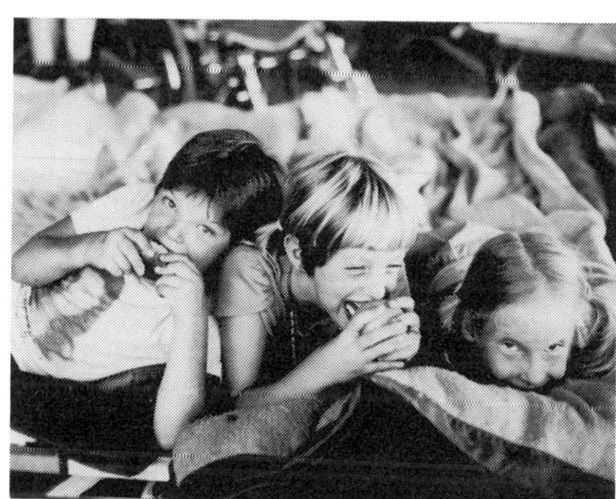

Parades sometimes were spontaneous at camp, and other times were planned (left). At right giggly campers had fun on a camp out.

signed on a unique open-air principle and furnished with an electric organ, comfortable bench-pews, and a little altar. Campers volunteered to hold the services.

At most any time of day a parade of comical sorts, an impromptu competition or race, or a burst of good fun would suddenly happen. These made happy and laughable memories. One time a number of campers rushed into the program office, hauled out the staffers, tied them to a tree, and sprayed them with shaving lotion. No member of the staff or counselor ever minded being the object of a joke. Their constant motto was: "Drop the dignity." The campers' motto was. "Expect the unexpected."

It only took a couple of days each session for the blind kids to join in on the fun in their own way, for the deaf to come in for their share of jokes, and for the mute to learn how easy it was to fully participate. They helped each other, and they had a keen sense of understanding so that no one felt left out.

If there was a way to do something fun, the Lions campers found it together. As long as there were kids and young people, there would be spontaneous fun. Lion campers sitting at one table in the dining hall might start singing, then challenge the other tables to do better. At least several times a week there would be a crutch or wheelchair race, a great favorite among the handicapped children. Said one boy, "I never had anyone at home to race with me. No one else is in a wheelchair."

Fun happened in the bunkhouses, which was given a special theme at the beginning of the session. Decorations were made, and songs were composed. There was much healthy rivalry between bunkhouses, not only centered about the various themes, but in striving to win cleanest bunkhouse honors. At one summer session an older boys' bunkhouse selected the theme of "Male chauvinist pig," and at one lunch meal, they all arrived wearing fake pig noses. Sometimes there were brother-sister wings, and they planned activities together. Although the general camp program was well planned, there was plenty of time for creativity and imagination in every area of camp. When carnivals or talent shows were held, originality in costuming came shining through. Pajama parades were held, and trips to town for a movie or pizza were planned once in a while.

The camp staff realized that one of the most important things in daily living at camp was plenty of good, wholesome food! Kids get hungry in the outdoors; most gained several pounds at camp. They ate anything and everything, said the cooks who were picked for their love of children and expertise in their jobs. Thomas Andrysiak, a graduate of culinary art, who was the food service manager in 1989, used various methods to insert fun into mealtime. One week he put up a sign that said the kids had to "smile for dessert"; friends read this important message to their blind buddies. Most of them laughed out loud that summer because Andrysiak stood behind the counter making faces. He picked the children to ring the bell for each of the three meals. Andrysiak would hold the boy or girl up high so he or she could reach the pull chord. When asked how many times the bell was rung for the meals, Andrysiak said, "Until I get tired holding him." Kitchen supervisors at the Lions camp worked up a page of suggested menus for the camp outs and encouraged the wing leaders to let the kids pick the menu. Snacks were always ready for the campers: mid-morning, mid-afternoon, bedtime. The children had choices of milk or orange juice, with perhaps cookies or chips.

The last night of each two-week camp session was the exciting and emotion-packed Awards Night, which was attended often by as many as a thousand persons, including campers, counselors, staff, families and Lions. The latter were as excited as anyone, waiting to hear if the camper they sponsored won a special award. Actually, every camper received an award. These were given at a pre-Awards Night wing party. The formal awards ceremony at the amphitheatre featured a program of special introductions, stunts, songs, a few brief speeches, and the presentation of the Best Camper Award to one boy and one girl. These were selected by vote of the counselors. The Texas City Lions Club, which donated money to build and maintain the miniature golf course, sponsored a golf tourney at each session and provided trophies for the low scorer at each session. Every activity department also gave awards. Anticipation was very high beginning at sunup on Awards Day. For the long march to the amphitheatre after supper, campers dressed in their best camp clothes, including the light blue camp T-shirts emblazed with Indian "coup feathers." Coup feathers were given campers or wings for outstanding performance. A feather was like a pat on the back for a good deed.

Campers usually felt happy with themselves and their accomplishments at Awards Night, but they all seemed sad to be leaving the special hilltop. The atmosphere at the amphitheatre elicited both laughter and tears. Some children walked with awkward crutches or in weighty braces; many rolled in wheelchairs; some had never seen the sunset, and others had never heard their friends' voices. Said Executive Director Crawford, "At Awards Night each face beams radiantly as the camper struggles down the path to receive a special award. You see only a child, just like any other child, with a soul, perfect, beautiful, and you share the exquisite joy of each child's happiness."

This would be the last time the campers would be forming the Friendship Circle until next year. Families, Lions, and others at the ceremony joined hands in the Friendship Circle. Then, for the final time the camp song was sung:

> Each campfire lights anew,
> the flame of friendship true;
> the joys we've had in knowing you
> will last a whole life through;
> and as the embers fade away,
> we wish we could ever stay,
> but since we cannot have our way,
> we'll come again some other day.

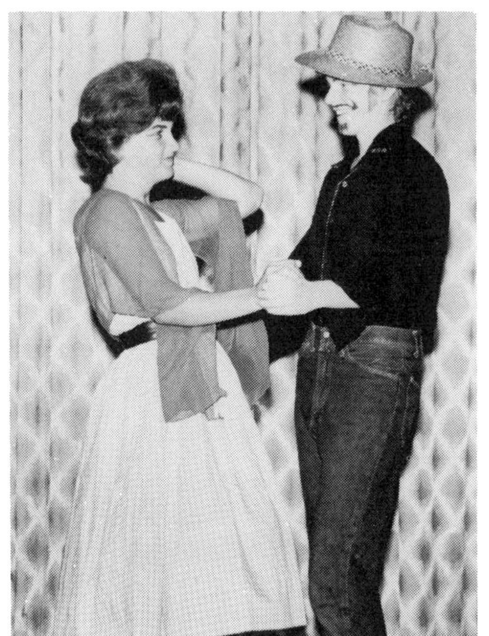

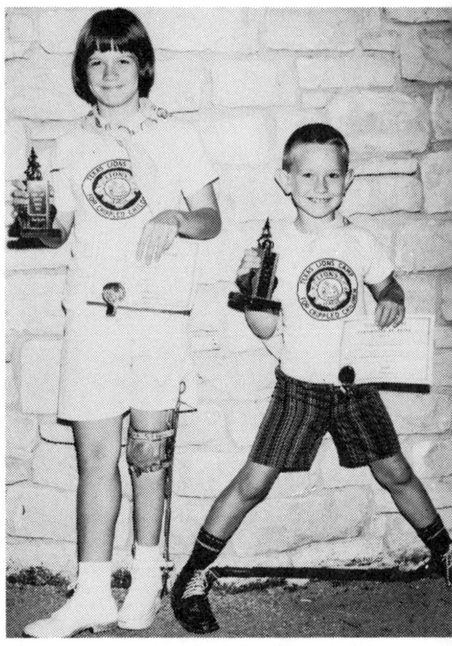

Teen-age campers at left were mute, which in no way affected their enjoyment of dancing. Climax of camp was Awards Night. At right, two children, voted by counselors as Best Campers of that session, proudly displayed awards.

Wrote one parent:

> I would like to take this time to say thank you for the love and care you gave to my son. What each of you do for our children is such a special thing. This was our first year with the camp and I hope there will be more as I see how this time has benefitted Zach. The Awards Night was delightful and there were tears in my eyes as I watched how you made each of these children feel so special.

Fourteen golden days which had just passed for these kids would make a loving chapter in their books of life. Each one would hope all during the coming year that the Lions back home would come calling with an application form that would reserve them a place again next year on the hilltop so close to heaven.

— Chapter 5 —

"A New World Unfolds"

"Just think of all the other kids who would like to be in our place."
— A Camper

Joshua's teacher announced the first English assignment for the fall semester: "Write a theme on what you did on your summer vacation." Eleven-year-old Roberto had never been on a vacation, because his family was poor. This particular summer he had been selected by a Lions Club in his city to attend their camp for handicapped children. He qualified because he lost both legs in a tractor accident when he was five years old. Since that time, Joshua had propelled himself around on a scooter board which an older brother made for him.

During the short two-week camping session at the Lions facility near Kerrville, he was taken into a swimming pool for the first time in his life, and he learned how to swim. He spent one night in a tent on a hill where he could see nothing above him but the sky. The Lions camp had fitted him with artificial legs and taught him to use them, so when he met his parents in El Paso, he was standing up and wearing his first pair of full-length jeans. Joshua began his

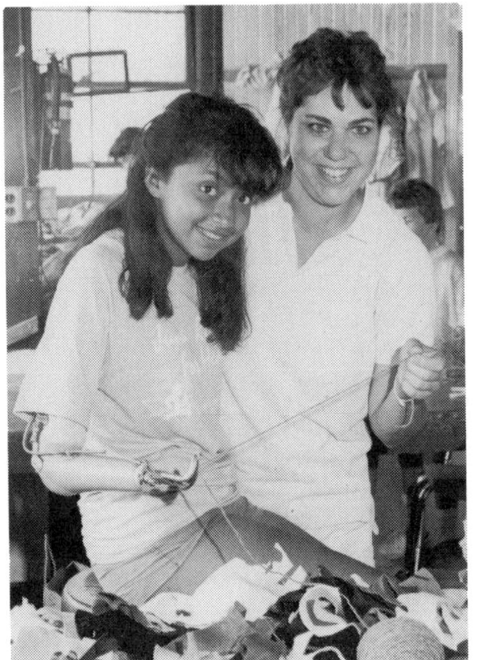

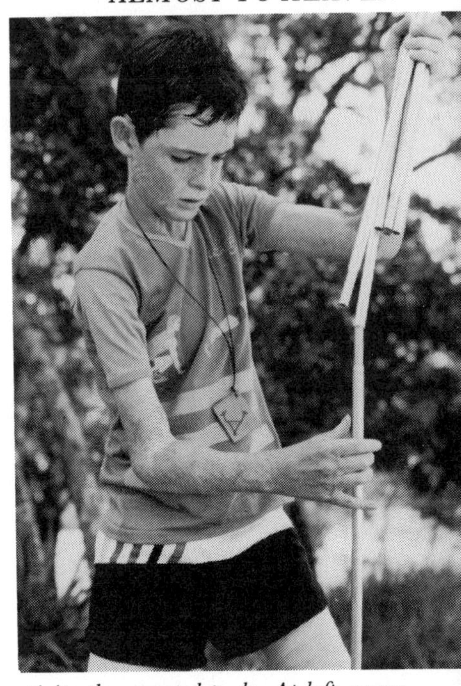

Handicaps did not keep campers from any activity they wanted to do. At left, young girl and counselor worked in arts and crafts. Camper at right concentrated on putting up a tent.

English theme with "I became just like all the other kids on my summer vacation. I got legs and learned how to walk."

For unknown reasons, Rhonda had never been able to speak. Therapists could not draw words from her; parents' attempts also failed. She received a free trip to the Lions camp one summer, and became friends with Jack, who was paralyzed from the waist down and who lived in a wheelchair. She pushed him to various camp activity sites, but sometimes just walked beside the chair as he navigated. Jack talked incessantly. There was communication between the boy and girl known only by them, but he wanted to hear Rhonda say words. He did not give up. All day long, as the pair went from class to dining hall to bunkhouses, he begged her to speak. He looked deep into her eyes and made her watch him form words. She finally, hesitantly, made an effort to talk. Other campers helped, urging her to talk, and trying to include her in the singing sessions. Before the end of the two-week camping period, Rhonda was saying short sentences, shyly giggling after each one.

Jack and the other campers clapped when she spoke. When Rhonda arrived home, she said, "Hi, Mom." Rhonda's English theme was entitled "I learned how to talk on my summer vacation."

One day counselors at camp noticed the wind had picked up a bit, so they planned to fly kites with the children. Anita was deaf and mute. She learned the two-handed art of kite-flying quickly, but had a hard time expressing her delight at the fun. She needed her hands for sign language. Next time her counselor looked at her, she saw Anita holding the string with her teeth, using one hand to jostle the string and the other hand to yell and laugh. Her theme paper was headed by the words, "How I learned to do things for myself on my summer vacation."

Mac was an unhappy boy when he went to the Lions camp. He had been unhappy all his life. Born with congenital malformation of legs and arms, his legs were very short and he only walked slowly and with effort. His arms were flippers adjoining his shoulders. He had never had a playmate. When his parents went to town, they left him on the back seat of the car. At first, he just grunted at passersby at camp and sat on the sidelines as he had always done. He observed the other boys and girls, in various states of handicaps, doing fun things. Mac could not help himself. He wanted to have fun, too, so he gradually entered the orbit of players. By the end of camp, he had become another problem for the counselors; he was loud and boisterous. He would stand up on a step stool after dishes were cleared away and loudly sing a song of his own creation. "Listen to me," he would say. One boy in English class wrote about the high mountains he had seen on his summer vacation; Mac wrote about the high mountains he had moved on his summer vacation. Mac made friends for the first time in his life on the Lions hilltop.

Doris heard the older girls talking about summer fun at a church camp, and she couldn't wait until she was eight years old and could go, too. When she was seven she had polio and faced a lifetime of wearing a tightfitting body brace and braces on both legs. Church camp was out because it only accepted physically "normal" children. One day a member of the local Lions club knocked at her door and talked to her parents. Doris went to the largest and most innovative Lions camp in the world at Kerrville, where she left her braces on the banks of the pool and learned to

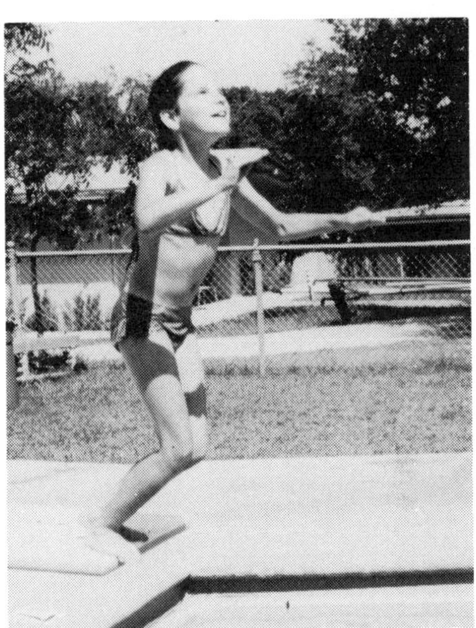
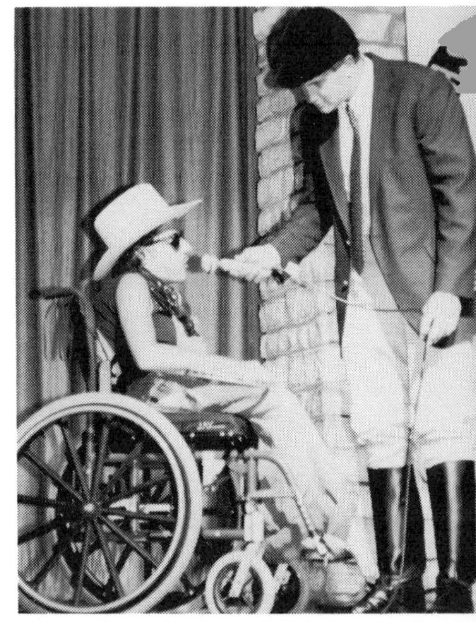

Blind swimmer at left had total faith in her ability in the water, a newly learned skill taught so carefully by counselors. Horsemanship supervisor, far right, interviewed camper at a stunt night.

swim. Her theme was centered around discovering a new life for herself on her summer vacation.

Danny was born with a withered right hand. He would not allow anyone to touch it, and he tried to hide it. Danny went to the Lions camp, played games designed to strengthen muscles and confidence. When he went home, his parents were amazed that, instead of hiding the hand, he extended it. He knew that "On my summer vacation I learned to shake hands."

Gilbert was so physically handicapped that he lived in his wheelchair and had to be fed and dressed. He had an active mind and a clear, distinctive voice. At the Lions camp he was selected to play the part of Judge Roy Bean in a stunt night skit. It took two others to complete the Judge Bean character — one to push Gilbert around on the stage, and another to hold the script and turn the pages. The skit was going along successfully when a breeze whipped out one of the pages to the script. Instantly a little boy on the front seat retrieved the page and handed it up, saying, "Here it is, Judge." Gilbert was a stage star on his summer vacation.

Emmett did not have any arms; he was born with hands where his arms should have been and they didn't meet. At the Lions camp he made a wallet for his brother after an arts and crafts counselor rigged a device to hold the leather so Emmett could lace the pieces together, using his teeth and one hand at a time. Emmett won the honor camper award for his two-week stay at the camp.

After Juan lost a leg in an automobile accident, he became a recluse, but local Lions persuaded him to go to camp. He decided he would not participate. Then he saw a counselor, who had an artificial leg, teaching some of the boys how to play soccer. Juan asked the counselor: "You mean you can run?" Juan learned to run, too. He also learned to dance and had his first date at a camp party. He played soccer at his school in the fall. Commented the smiling counselor, "Oh, Juan is just a normal little jerk." And Juan wrote a theme for his English class about how he learned to forget self-pity on his vacation.

These were the kinds of children who went to the hilltop camp in Central Texas. When the sun spread its first morning rays over the woods, these were the children that interrupted the serenity and kept the place buzzing until they fell asleep at night, too tired to think of limitations or self-pity. The Lions program was keyed to the goal of teaching them self-reliance, consideration of others and development of talents and abilities. Buddy looked after buddy and teamed up to help each other. The spirit spilled over into their home life, and later into adulthood.

Polio victim Judy went to camp several years, though paralyzed from the waist down. She became a champion swimmer and went home to win medals there, too. She and her mother were active in the National Foundation for Infantile Paralysis and spent a lot of time giving hope to parents and victims. Roberto, who spent four years at the Lions camp, had been a baseball star in his hometown when both legs were cut off too high to be able to wear artificial limbs. He learned to make his own dollies, or skateboards, for mobility; and as a teen-ager he was a major organizer of little league baseball teams. He became helper to his father who was a roofer. Roberto could climb ladders with agility, and he loved working on rooftops; they reminded him of Inspiration Point. He said the Lions camp, together with the other handicapped children, made him think of his capabilities rather than disabilities, which brought new dimensions to his life.

Camp staffers tried to satisfy each child's natural desire to be a part of things. They bridged the gap between a former isolated and unimportant existence to a life full of promise and productivity. For many of the children the Lions camp was the first place they felt really happy with themselves. Overprotection of parents was erased with experiences in group living. Said one counselor, "Handicapped kids can do almost anything they want to at camp. They begin to look around and accept themselves for what they really are and really can do." Most were very nervous at first, but competition gave them a willingness to try hard, then they earned victories, no matter how small. Camp Executive Director Glenn Crawford said "we try to instill in them the idea that they can live with their problems; and not only that, but they can live happily with them."

Seven-year-old Agnes spent forty-five minutes making her way from her bunkhouse to the dining hall, but she would not let anyone help her. Scotty wore his Cub Scout cap everywhere, even in the swimming pool; and when he was on the camp-outs, he slipped marshmallows under the cap. George was a camp clown, and did tricks and balancing acts with his crutches. Elmer claimed the fanciest hot-rod wheelchair in camp and challenged others to races. One camper, Ellen, became so fast on her wheels that when she went back to school, they presented her with a driver's license in a special ceremony. Other campers bugged Ben to tell them the jokes he read in his braille book. Another blind camper was called the "Mr. Magoo of Unit Two" because he ran into a tree one time and said, "Excuse me, tree, I thought you were somebody else." Every morning Cecile asked the counselor, "Shall I wear my leg this morning?"

Siblings who had attended camp together included boy triplets who were blind at birth; twins John and Paula; Kent, eleven, and his sister, Cherie, ten; Danny, a polio victim, age eleven, and his seven-year-old sister, Cheryl, who had cerebral palsy. These were the children of the Texas Lions camp who wished the summer would last forever. Some children had been to camp for as many as seven or eight years, until they were seventeen years old. However, when Lions sent applications for campers each spring, the camp considered new campers over former campers because it tried to

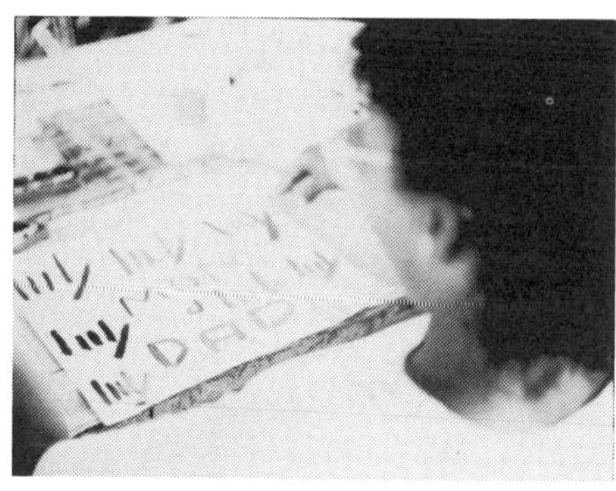

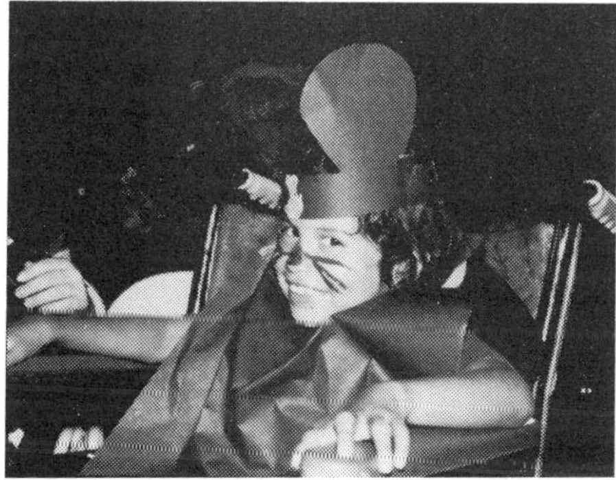

At left, hearing-impaired camper made her first painting for her parents. Signs on the painting said "love." At right was a happy, costumed camper.

give as many children as possible at least one opportunity to experience camping. One mother said "I don't know what I'm going to do while Camarie's gone to camp. Our lives revolve around our children." But another mother said she knew Carolyn would be fine; "I'm the one who is apprehensive." When Bill returned from a camp session, tanned and heavier, his mother said that he felt he could do things other boys could do. "The camp made an entirely different person out of Bill." Parents of Kevin called the Lions camp experience an excellent way for him to learn to function away from them, while another couple said they believed that most of all, "momma and daddy learned that Jared could get along without us." For many campers the camp vacation was the first time they had been away from home except for the times they were in the hospital.

Steven's mother said "If it were not for the Lions Camp, our son would probably be dead." His legs were strapped to a brace that severely limited his movement. He had had several operations, and had no desire to get out of bed. He said he was "tired of being laughed at and tired of being cut on." One year later, after a session at the Lions camp, Steven was able to run and was excited about all the things he was going to do with his life. For many of the children, it was the first time to make a bed, help prepare a meal, or share a secret with a buddy.

When counselors elected best boy and girl camper of each session they took into consideration the child's leadership qualities, enthusiasm, appearance, personality, interests in all camp programs, personal cleanliness, social adjustment, eating habits, willingness to cooperate, observance of camp regulations, adherence to health and safety for self and others; and then they considered ability and skills.

One year counselors polled campers, asking such questions as "What was your favorite activity?" to which one little girl answered, "I really like Artery." When asked what they learned at camp, one replied, "many things" and another said he learned "to be independent, not to be scared and not to be homesick." One boy learned not to hit other people. The Lions Camp record for rehabilitating handicapped boys and girls rated high, but the program staffs, through the years, admitted that they did not hit bulls eyes every time. Sometimes behavioral problems were too great, and the child had to be sent home. Other times it might have been that the child's handicaps were too great for the Camp's limited staff, and the Lions who sponsored the child did not realize it.

Among the many physical disabilities acceptable for a camper were amputee, blind/vision impaired, burns, cancer/tumor, cerebral palsy, deaf/hard of hearing, deaf/blind, juvenile rheumatoid arthritis, Legg-Perthes, muscular dystrophy, mute, partial paralysis, polio, rickets, sclerosis, certain strokes. Mentally handicapped children were not accepted; campers must have had an IQ of seventy or above. Other facilities existed for children with mental handicaps. Other ineligible conditions were hemophilia, osteogenesis imperfecta, contagious diseases, emotionally disturbed, bedfast, autistic. According to the Texas Department of Health, the five most prevalent conditions among the handicapped children which they serve are congenital malformation of the heart or great vessels, cerebral palsy, otitis media, cleft palate or cleft lip, and spina bifida. Campers were between seven and seventeen years of age.

Children were grouped by age and sex, but not by handicaps,

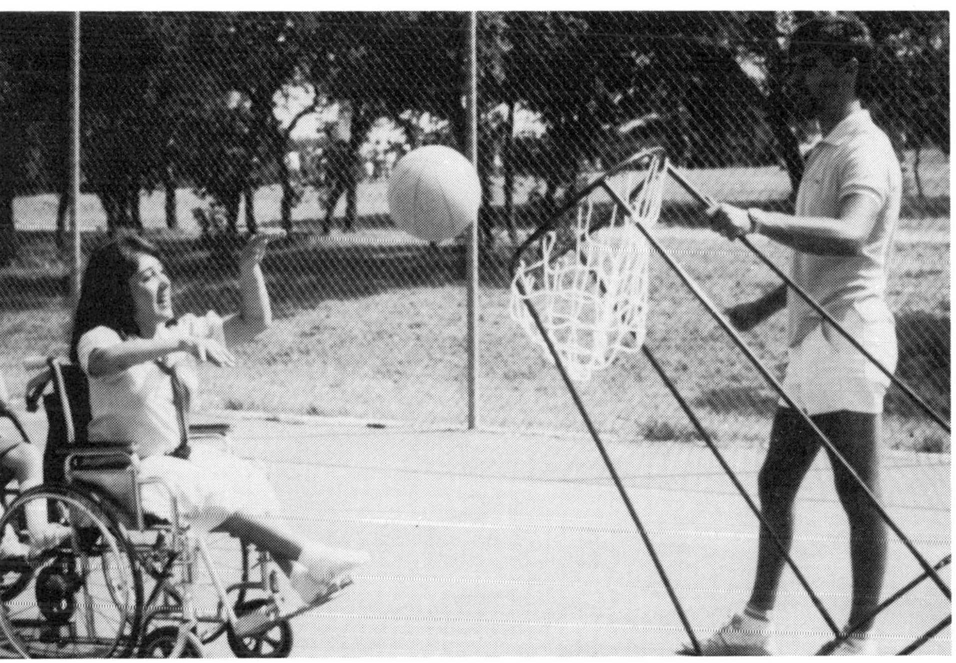

Everyone was a winner at Texas Lions Camp!

so they became aware at camp of the many different problems of handicapped kids. Soon, staffers found, the least important thing about the campers were their handicaps. The days were busy for everyone; reveille awoke the children at 6:30, and breakfast was at 7:00 o'clock. Then began bunkhouse checks, assemblies, activity classes, free time, lunch, rest period, snacks, activities, and supper at 6:00 P.M., followed by surprise entertainments in the evening and "lights out" at 9:00 P.M. when "taps" was played.

After reveille every morning, one of the camper units was in charge of raising the flag while the national anthem was played over the loud speaker. A neighborhood problem arose one summer. Crawford received a telephone call from the nearby Veterans' Hospital. It seemed that the bugle which sounded reveille was heard loud and clear at the hospital. The nurses were having problems when some hospitalized veterans awoke and stood at attention beside their beds. The nurses did not want their patients awaking at 6:30 A.M.

During one of the summer sessions the Kerrville Catholic Church held a special program to which the Catholic campers were invited. In order to go, these campers were allowed to eat supper early. Campers worked up amazing appetites, and one hungry little boy tugged on a counselors sleeve and asked, "When do the Baptists get to eat?" to which she replied, "When the Presbyterians eat."

It was not always the grandiose things that campers remembered. They cherished their associations with other children like themselves and were proud of little things like learning to put on their braces, lace their shoes, climb on the top bunk, clean the bathrooms, and open and shut doors. They liked being told, "You can do it. Now get in there and clean up the bunkhouse!" In their hometowns, they could not compete with the other children at their schools, and no one expected them to do it. One program director said the biggest handicap the Lions children endured was having friends and relatives who did everything for them. At the Lions camp they shined; attention was on each of them; they set goals and reached them.

The final day of each two-week camping session was the most important day of all. Every camper received an award. The first day of camp ran a close second to most important. Concluding that first day was the traditional Friendship Circle where each boy and girl threw a wish stick into the campfire. Campers were asked to bring a little stick to the activity. At the end of announcements and songs, the campers came, one by one, to the edge of the fire, made a wish and blew it into the stick, then threw it into the fire. An old Indian legend said the smoke carried the wish all over the world, making it come true.

For many years, every camper received a bandana at the end of the session on which were stamped his or her honors and medals won. Campers later received certificates suitable for framing. All went home with a blue and white camp T-shirt.

Counselors, staffers and Lions call the camp children "kids." They are like all other kids, said a staff member, but where else would the heroine of a skit be on crutches and the hero in a wheelchair? Where else would a camper complain that a deaf buddy "never hears when it comes to work time?"

These are the unique and lovable campers at the Texas Lions hilltop. These are the kids who want to be just like all the other kids.

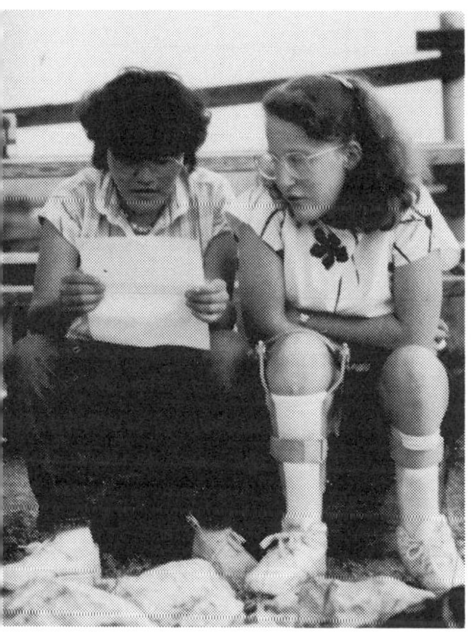

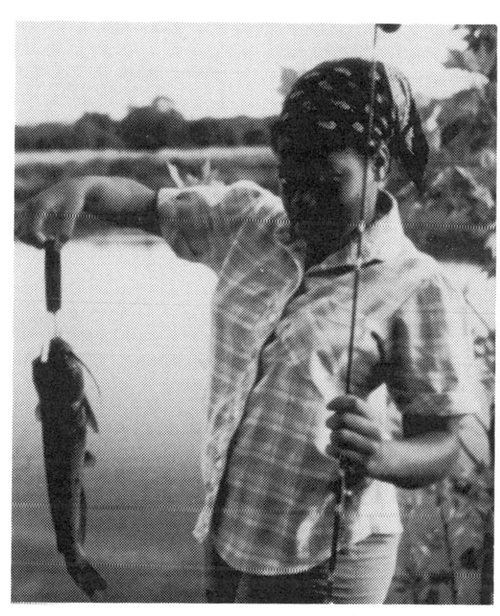

At left, letters from home were important at camp. . . . "I got a big 'un!" smiled young angler at camp pond.

— Chapter 6 —

"The Invisible Disease"

"Don't feel sorry for these kids. Just marvel at their ability to make the most out of life."

— Richard Morehead, *Dallas Morning News*

A Lion visited one of the class sessions during the final summer session at the Texas Lions Camp. He was surprised to hear the teen-agers asking such questions as: Will I be able to marry? Can I have children? Is it contagious? Can it cause a natural abortion if I get pregnant?

These were questions that "normal-looking" kids with an invisible or hidden disease wanted answered. These were kids with diabetes who were attending the Lions camp session especially set up for them. The visitor wondered why this group of boys and girls who looked so normal were attending a camp for the handicapped.

Such visitor, evidently, had never seen a diabetic with a seizure or in a coma which could be fatal. He had never seen young eyes that were fading possibly into blindness. He had never seen a youngster with such serious diabetes that there was a possibility of losing a limb with gangrene. According to medical statistics, a dia-

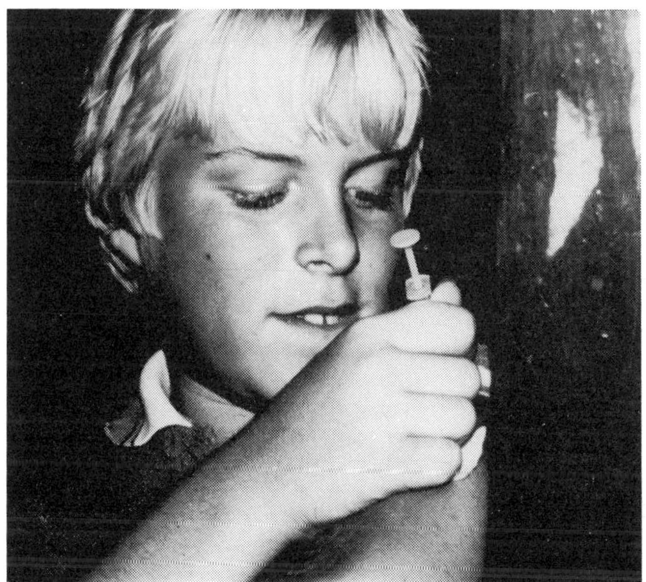

Diabetic camper learned to give his own shots.

betic can expect his life to be cut, possibly, by one-third because of this dread disease for which there is no known cure.

It was not hidden to these campers. It was in the forefront of their daily lives. "Will I still have friends, even tho' I can't eat pizza?" went through their confused minds. Is it true that I can't have any sweets? What will happen between me and my boyfriend; will he not like me any more?" These very important medical and social problems were addressed at the Texas Lions Camp for Diabetic Children. They were handled by an expert professional team of doctors and nurses specializing in diabetes plus a group of well-trained camp counselors.

Directors of both the medical and camp staffs assured prospective campers that there would be careful coordination on the Lions scenic hilltop between a happy balance of exercise and activities plus medical care. Teaching methods were utilized which maximize learner involvement and peer interaction. No formal lectures are held; instead the techniques were used that made medical sessions lively, including playacting, visual presentations, touching and seeing. For the youngest campers, beginning at age seven, games, puppets and other playtime activities were some of the tools for education. Camp itself was conducive for learning. It was quiet, comfortable, informal and uninterrupted except maybe for the call of a bird or scurry of a rabbit.

These specialized camp sessions for children with diabetes sought to teach them to choose their diets, test their blood sugar levels, give their own shots, and then balance all this with their normal activities.

Carlos, age nine, had gone to the Lions camp knowing only how to do the urine test. He had been nervous doing that. The idea of giving himself insulin shots terrified Carlos. Counselors and medical staffers worked with him in learning relaxation techniques and encouraged him with soothing consolation and determined patience. When camp was over that year, Carlos went home able to give his own daily insulin shots. One positive learning experience which convinced Carlos that giving himself shots wasn't too bad was watching seven-year-old Donny in the next bunk give himself three shots a day. Carlos needed only one. Said Carlos's mother, "The whole camp is fantastic, and being with other diabetics is great. Carlos knows no one at home his age with diabetes, and knowing and seeing how others act and deal with it is the best thing for him."

For a few summer days, the Lions camper entered a community where the non-diabetic was in the minority. This brought an amazing realization for a child. All around were others with diabetes and, surprisingly, they all looked normal. This was an emotionally satisfying discovery. At the diabetes camp the child's social isolation was decreased and he was put among peers with whom to share and compare.

What is diabetes? It is usually an inherited disease which prevents the body from using sugar normally. Sugar is the substance bodies use as their major source of energy. A hormone (insulin) that a body should make is missing or deficient. Sugar can't be broken down effectively, and the cells of the body "starve." Fuel for the cells is usually a substance called glucose, which is necessary for the body to function. The brain and all parts of the nervous system *must* have glucose or food to function. Injections of insulin enables the body to break the single sugars into usable components taken throughout the body in the blood stream.

Diabetes is usually a familial disease, and the majority of peo-

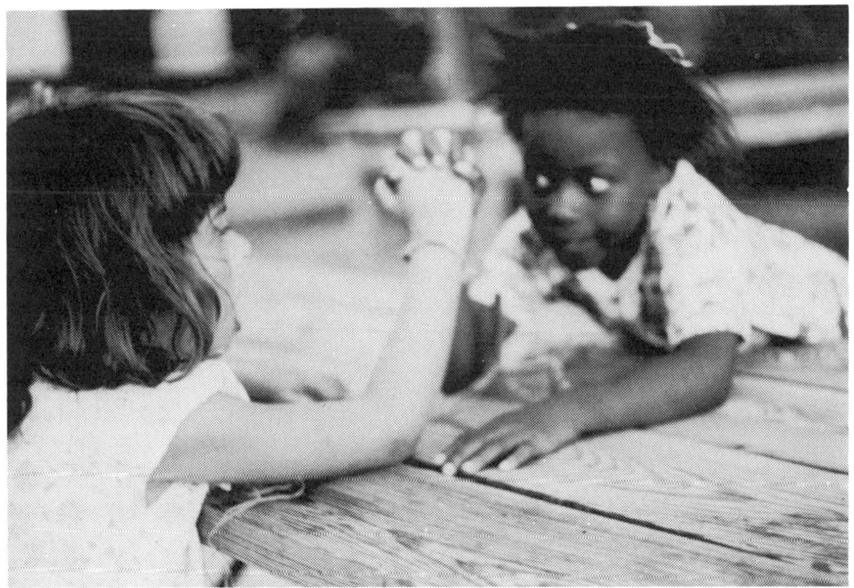

All kinds of fun kept campers busy all day!

ple develop "Type II Diabetes" after the age of forty and may not require insulin injections. Diabetes in the young, "Type I," is somewhat rare and requires insulin injections. Only Type I diabetic children can attend the camp. One parent wrote that her child found camp made living with diabetes just a little easier because she saw she wasn't alone with her troubles. She could share her problems and thoughts related to diabetes with others at camp. She also learned a great deal about herself and made many new friends. "I really do appreciate the great care and love you gave my child at the Lions camp."

The Texas Lions League was founded in 1949 when polio was striking the children of the nation, so it was set up for "crippled children." In a few years terminology changed to replace "crippled" with "handicapped." Diabetes severely handicaps its victims. It can be a killer. After Salk found the miraculous vaccine against polio and the disease almost disappeared, the Lions looked around for children with other types of disabilities. They found many. They also found children who had diabetes. Texas Lionism again raised its understanding head.

Camping is described by the American Camping Association as "sustained experience which provides a creative, recreational and educational opportunity in group living in the out-of-doors. It utilizes trained leadership and the resources of natural surroundings to contribute to each camper's mental, physical, social and spiritual growth."

Although the ACA requirements were tough, the Lions camp was accredited from its inception. Actually, these guidelines were only the starting point for the League's camp. They imposed upon themselves a much stricter second set of guidelines and carried out intensive specialized training for personnel because their campers were children who were physically or visually impaired, or had hearing or speech disabilities. Every staffer studied each of these special problems so they could knowledgeably understand and help the children.

When the camp for diabetics was formed, yet a third set of guidelines was needed, so all personnel were required to have a knowledge of this disease. The Lions Camp was endorsed by the American Diabetes Association, which had its own requirements for accreditation — a fourth set of guidelines.

The diabetic camp objectives included the following: to provide an enjoyable recreational camping experience in a safe and healthy environment, to enable children with diabetes to meet and associate with other children with similar problems, to help children with diabetes to learn more about their disorder so that they could be better able to control the problems of living with a chronic illness, to teach diabetics independence and self-discipline in the approach to their disease and their approach to life, and to provide an educational program for the parents which became an integral part of the overall program.

Said one parent: "Thanks for your generosity and concern for these kids. Please don't ever let anything interfere with the diabetic session. It is so important to these children and their parents." Another wrote that no price could be put on the camp's value to both the children and the parents.

As with the camp for crippled children, no diabetic child or his family paid for the stay at camp; they were guests of the Texas Lions Clubs and friends who gave tax deductible donations.

The first diabetic camp in Texas was held as a one-week session in the summer of 1959 on the site of Camp Manison in

Friendswood, near Houston. It was organized under the auspices of the Houston and Gulf Coast Diabetes Association, and one of its primary founders was Dr. C. W. Daeschner, chairman of the Department of Pediatrics, the University of Texas Medical Branch at Houston. Nineteen children attended that summer when the ground was laid for a long and productive future course.

Dr. Luther B. Travis, also of the UT medical branch in Galveston, became associated with the Friendswood camp the next year. He was appointed medical director in 1964. When the Texas Lions League entered the picture in 1971, it assumed partial and then full financial responsibility for the camp. Dr. Travis remained as medical director. The Lions camp was the only diabetes camp in the nation which was fully supported by an organization such as the Lions.

Dr. Travis was recognized as one of the foremost diabetic medical directors in the nation. The Lions League believed its camp had "the best care of any in the world." Dr. Travis, who was professor of pediatrics at the UT school in Galveston, also was director of their divisions of nephrology and diabetes and was director of the Children's Diabetes Management Center. Since diet was so important for persons with diabetes, Dr. Travis brought with him each summer a special diabetes dietitian.

Dr. Travis said the camp provided a fine experience for professionals specializing in pediatrics or diabetes because here they dealt with the children and their disabilities on a twenty-four hour basis for two straight weeks.

In addition to a two-day camp workshop in Galveston in early spring each year, medical staffers received another two days of training just prior to the camp's opening. For the medical staff, Dr. Travis prepared an inch-thick manual, also used at his Children's Diabetes Management Center. His staff also thoroughly learned the inch-thick general staff manual prepared by the Lions camp which all regular counselors knew. Under "Camp Rules" in the medical guideline book, the orders were: "We, the medical staff, are guests at the camp and will abide by the rules and regulations of the camp. If staying in bunkhouse with kids, we will abide by cabin rules."

Every diabetic camper's doctor back home received a detailed report of the child's progress, problems and activities while at the facility. The professional team felt it could help educate many phy-

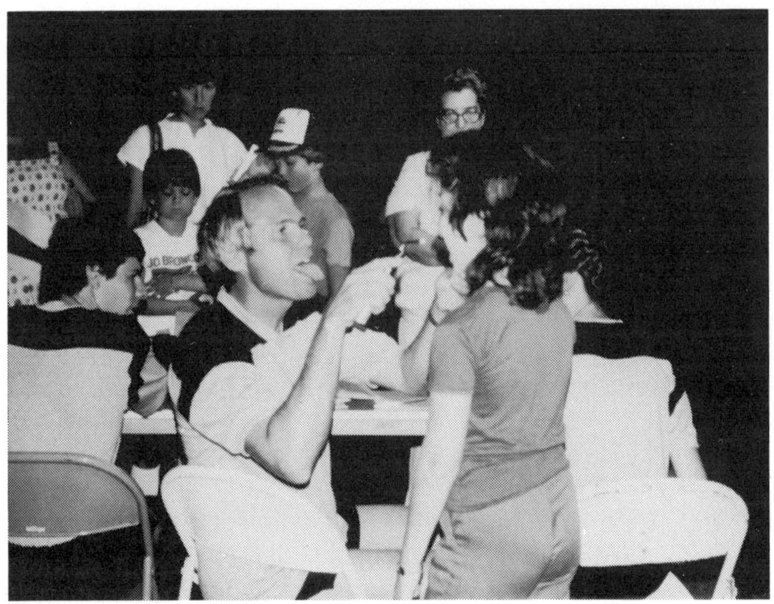

Doctor who was diabetic specialist gave medical checkup during first day.

sicians in Texas because the team had been in a unique position of monitoring the diabetic from sun up to sun down in living, working, and playing conditions.

A medical counselor sat at every eating table, casually explaining about some of the foods which were served. Counselors checked all snacks, and explained why some were acceptable for a diabetic and why some were not.

The horrible words, "no junk foods," might have a devastating effect on a diabetic who thought his friend did not call him because, with his disease, he was no longer acceptable. The Lions camp program was designed to present information that would enable the camper to make decisions about himself. The major goal was to assist the diabetic in achieving maturity in a healthy and productive manner. The camp showed them, while they were having fun, that they can live happy, normal lives by following good health practices.

Like at all camps around the world, homesickness was sometimes a problem, which most often was of short duration with correct solutions, but it could occur in any age boy or girl. The staff at the Lions camp looked for a friend for the homesick camper first. They picked someone the camper could trust and who was firm in reinforcing camp as a fun, rewarding place. Generally this friend was on the program staff; but at the camp for diabetics, the medical staff backed him up with intervention help. In dealing with homesickness, the Lions staffers believed it was best not to be overly protective, overly concerned, or overly helpful. With the diabetic, a medical staffer would first rule out signs of hypoglycemia in the homesick child, checking blood sugar and symptoms in their behavior which might accelerate the disease. Homesickness was a "stressor" and might produce significant hyperglycemia and even Ketonuria. Both were serious. Hyperglycemia was high level of blood sugar, as opposed to hypoglycemia which was decreased sugar in blood, and Ketonuria was the condition of having too much acetone in the urine.

No camper with diabetes and homesickness at the Lions camp ever reached a serious stage. All staffers were trained to overcome this emotional experience as soon as possible. Much of the time by the end of camp a once homesick child was the one who cried when he had to leave. A number adjusted so well that they were selected to receive the coveted Distinguished Camper Award.

From 1971 until 1973 the Lions sponsored the camp at Friendswood, but in 1973 it split the sites, holding one diabetic camp at the Kerrville site. Then in 1980 all sessions were held in the Hill Country, one at the Lions camp and one at nearby Camp Rio Vista in Ingram. Beginning in 1986 all sessions of the diabetic camp were put under the one "parent" roof on the Lions hilltop. One session of the diabetic camp was held for the younger children, and one for the older ones.

Their success depended on teamwork between the medical staff and the Lions camp. Policies and administration of the diabetic camp were under the direction of Glenn Crawford, executive director of the Texas Lions League. The League assured funding for all activities, both recreational and medical-educational; accommodations; and most of the supplies. Many pharmaceutical companies generously donated large amounts of necessary medical supplies.

Criteria for the camp medical staff included: interest or experience with children or adolescents, camping experience, interest or

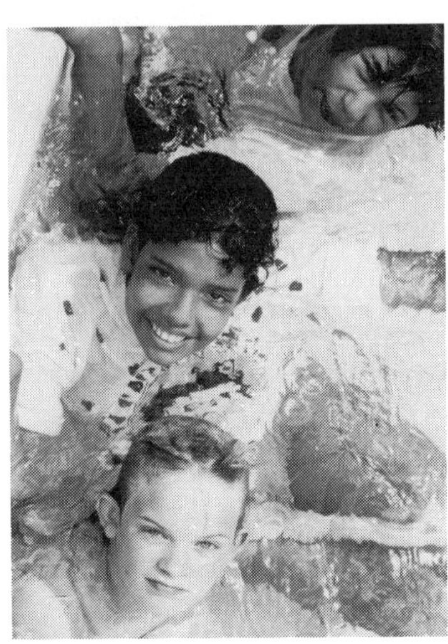

Water play and swimming lessons were always the most popular activity at Lions camp.

experience educating children or adolescents, knowledge of diabetes, ability to work in a team environment.

Dr. Richard Dusold, a pediatrician in Temple, Texas, was a diabetic camper at the Lions facility who returned as an aide, then as a counselor for two years. After he entered medical school, once more he returned to the diabetic camp on the medical staff. Dr. Dusold met his wife, Dianne, at the Lions Camp when both were on the medical team.

Five camp counselors were diabetic in the 1988 season, and all camp counselors attended the intensive two-day training course just before the diabetic sessions began. The counselors said they always remembered that when a kid said he felt low, they gave him a little sugar cube, then the medics could adjust his insulin intake later. At every activity area, a medic bought a complete kit for insulin-related emergencies and the counselors brought first aid kits.

Executive Director Crawford said it could be very frightening to witness a diabetic going into shock. The person might become pale and weak, looking "funny" in the eyes, and many times shaking all over. Orange juice, glucose, sugar cubes would bring them back with energy levels necessary for functioning. Sometimes, however, it was serious enough for a camper to be taken to the infirmary for three or four hours so that the medics could assist in bringing the camper's sugar level to normal requirements.

Lance began feeling very sad when he reached the age of seventeen and attended his last session of camp, so he signed up immediately to return as an aide at the diabetic camp. Lance said he was one of two diabetics in his high school. He and the other one, Wendy, for years ate their snacks together in the nurse's office every day. Lance said if his friends decided to go out for pizza, "I couldn't go." But he found his friends cared, because they began watching what he ate. When he became of dating age, Lance had already spent a few years at camp and had learned how to adjust his insulin doses before the dates so he could go out and eat and have fun, knowing the insulin would "kick in" at the right time. This knowledge was, in reality, a life-saver for him.

One summer at the Lions camp a diabetic boy in a wheelchair was the rowdiest on the grounds. Counselors and other campers played games with him, trying to keep him from speeding by in his wheelchair since he could roll faster than they could walk.

A medical aide who was a former camper always remembered the great, unsolved camp mystery. The diabetic boys had been on an overnight camp out; and in the middle of the night when everyone was finally asleep, rocks began hurdling down on them. That woke up everyone quick! They spread out with flashlights to find the rock-throwers, but they never did. At that time, the campers' thoughts and imaginations were on aliens and UFOs, and the mystery was never solved.

Throughout the days of the diabetic season, campers were being educated, whether they realized it or not. Little lessons in living with the disease came at mealtime, shot time, horseback riding time. One father said that "kids just don't listen to parents and doctors like they listen to camp staff and their peers. Thank you for all you've done and will do."

Growing up is hard enough for youngsters without the added complication of a life-threatening disease, wrote Bonnie Arnold in the *Kerrville Daily Times*.

> Each summer, diabetic children go to the Lions camp for a week to learn to cope with their sickness and the problems it adds

> to growing up." These are the seven- to seventeen-year-olds who would not be accepted at any other camp because of their hidden disease, she continued.
>
> All the traditional camping activities are offered, from swimming, softball, riflery and general crafts to karate, signing and mime, and creative dramatics. There are a total of 20 courses from which campers choose four for the week's activities. Older kids have already learned about medication and nutrition, so they are taught how to manage life with the disease. They learn to recognize danger signs and monitor their own precautions.

The article explained how campers and staffers discussed situations like dating, how to handle testing for blood sugar, and giving oneself a shot in public. The teens' education was more sophisticated than the younger diabetics' education. Camp Executive Director Glenn Crawford was quoted in the article as saying, "They are all average teenagers. They caused us to stay up late at night and we had all the summer romances any camp full of teenagers has, but we have to tell them about home life and sex education and pregnancy. Long term diabetes sometimes leads to loss of nerve function and sometimes impotence. They need to know about their lives and what they can do about it."

Many of the teens were concerned with genetics. Discussions on this came under the heading of life skills. Each summer the teen diabetics explored a different life skill. This age group also was old enough for college-level activities, such as karate, snorkeling, and primitive cookouts. The returned campers were very important and effective as role models for those campers on a first trip and for the younger ones. It was a "human" trait, said Crawford, for children of all ages and all bodies to want to try new skills and new experiences, especially if a role model is just ahead. That boosts their confidence.

Among the books that Dr. Travis wrote about diabetes was *An Instructional Aid on Juvenile Diabetes Mellitus.* It covered all areas of this hidden disease for the newcomer, parents and interested nonmedical people. It was printed in large type with color graphs and drawings and sounded as if the genial, laid-back doctor was right on the bench beside the Lions camp pool, talking easily to a camper.

Readers learned that, according to Dr. Travis, nothing could have been done to prevent the onset; diabetes will not go away and certain viruses may be connected with the onslaught of the disease.

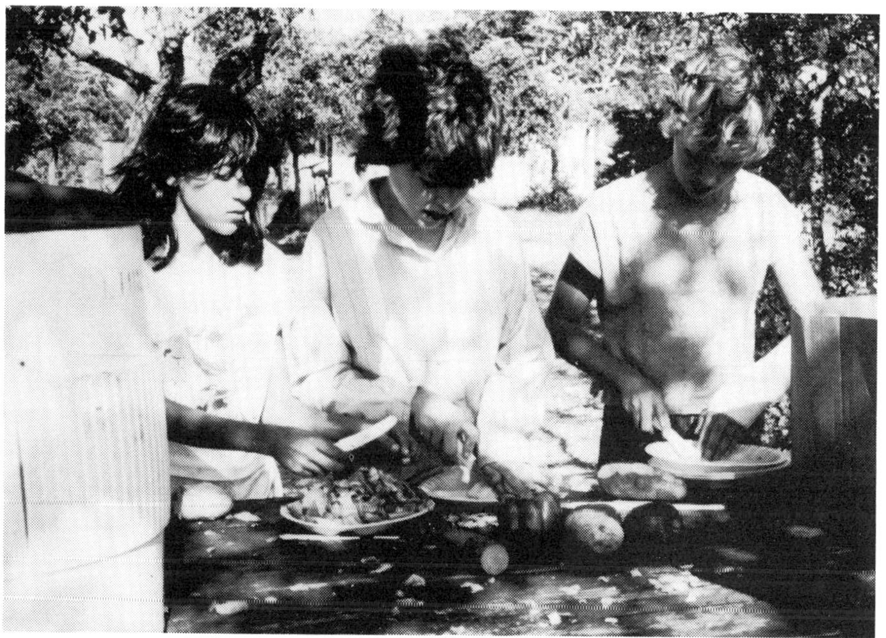

Cooking in the open on a camp out.

He named well-known persons who had to cope with diabetes: Mary Tyler Moore and Dan Rowan, TV stars; Ron Santo, Bobby Clarke, Billy Talbert, all famous athletes. He noted there were many others "out there."

Dr. Travis explained that the diabetic would not be able to ignore the disease but, with just a little extra attention to health, it would not significantly interfere with any aspect of normal life. Diabetes represents a little hardship, but keep it a "little one," he wrote.

Diabetic campers often asked Dr. Travis if having diabetes made a person feel different from his friends, to which he answered: "It probably does at times. In many ways, we are all different from one another. We're all individuals. This, by itself, says that we're all different from our friends. That's what makes each of us unique. But diabetes does make you more special and different. Because of your diabetes, you must pay more attention to food and diet, take insulin shots every day, monitor urine or blood sugars, get into a program of regular exercise, but with these exceptions, you should be able to look healthy, be healthy, do almost anything a non-diabetic can do, and live a long, happy, and productive life."

Dr. Travis and Director Crawford wanted their campers to go home feeling better about themselves and their diagnosed handicap. They hoped each one would be able to cope with problems that sometimes closed in on a diabetic and make them worse. In addition, Dr. Travis suggested that older diabetic children begin trying to help all they could in the diabetic field: join an association, help raise research money, talk to friends, talk to Congressmen, and visit persons recently diagnosed as diabetics to lend encouragement. The conclusion of his book had this to say: "You're going to do just fine. You really are. Have a nice life; you've earned it if you've worked with diabetes."

Parents of campers wrote continuously to Crawford. One begged the Lions to plan a two-week session for the diabetic camp. "Please let us parents know what we can do to make them two weeks. The parents sessions were very beneficial. It was Jamilyn's first time away from home and she loved it and wants to go back again next year. She feels 100 percent better about herself."

Diabetic children, with their hidden handicaps, were just like the children with handicaps that were readily recognized. They also had the same needs and desires. Daniel was in his seventh year at the Lions camp, which was his last year as he had turned seventeen. During every summer he had tried to jump off the big diving board. It was his ultimate goal. One day at free-swim in that last summer, he approached the big diving board. Using his greatest resolve, he got upon the board. Word passed quickly that Daniel was on the big diving board. Swimmers began treading water and watching; campers around the pool went to the fence; counselors rushed up; and staffers came out of the program office. Bodies lined the entire fenced area around the big pool. They were shouting, "Come on, Daniel. You can do it, Daniel. Yea, Daniel!"

Daniel did it! He jumped off the big diving board and swam to the side. He held his arm high and his hand made a victory sign.

It was every bit as emotionally stirring when Carlos, surrounded by buddies and counselors in his bunkhouse, experienced his greatest triumph. He had sat shaking every day, afraid to insert the insulin needle into his leg. Camp was almost over. He had lain on his bunk every night, praying that tomorrow he would be able to bring himself to do what the other kids did.

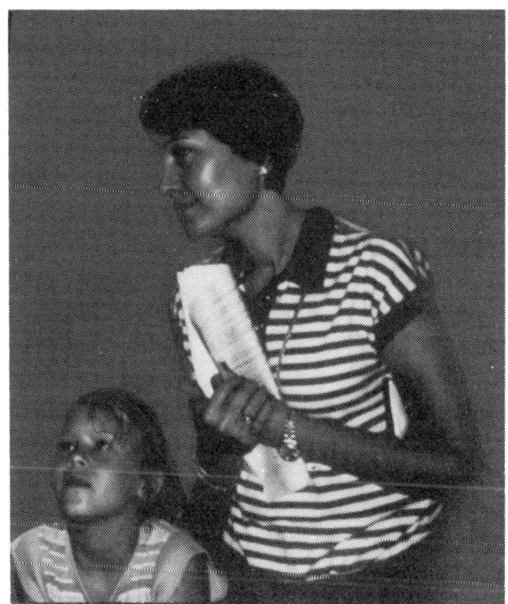

Parents and children learned about diabetes and how to cope with it.

"Come on, Carlos," yelled a friend, who was joined by others. "Yea, Carlos. You can do it!" By now even kids from other bunkhouses, hearing the noise, were around his cot, and so were counselors and several medics. "Carlos, get it in! Carlos, you can do it!"

A small, trembling hand slid in the needle. Carlos sighed with relief and his smile was as big as the Texas sky where the eagle flies. Carlos felt tall enough to reach almost to heaven.

— Chapter 7 —

"Keys to Camping: The Counselors"

"I'd rather go to the Lions Camp than Disneyworld."
— A camper

"What's the age of your counselors?" asked a visitor to the Texas Lions League Camp one day.

The good-looking young man, a waterfront counselor, started to answer. "Well, uh . . . let's see . . . I think most are college students, so . . . well, I guess about eighteen or nineteen years old to . . ." He glanced down the hill and saw Eddie jogging up it. Eddie was the oldest counselor at camp, with a tenure of thirty-two years. "Oops, make that eighteen years old to eighty-two years!"

Why did some college girls and boys spend every summer vacation as counselors at the Lions camp, then become sad when they graduated, got jobs and couldn't have summers free for camp anymore? "It's the kids. They get to you! I sure will miss my kids when I have to leave."

Camp Program Supervisor Oscar Lopez, who spent eight years as a counselor before he joined the staff in a full time capacity said about eight out of ten counselors returned as many years as possible. A plus for the counselors were the things they learned at

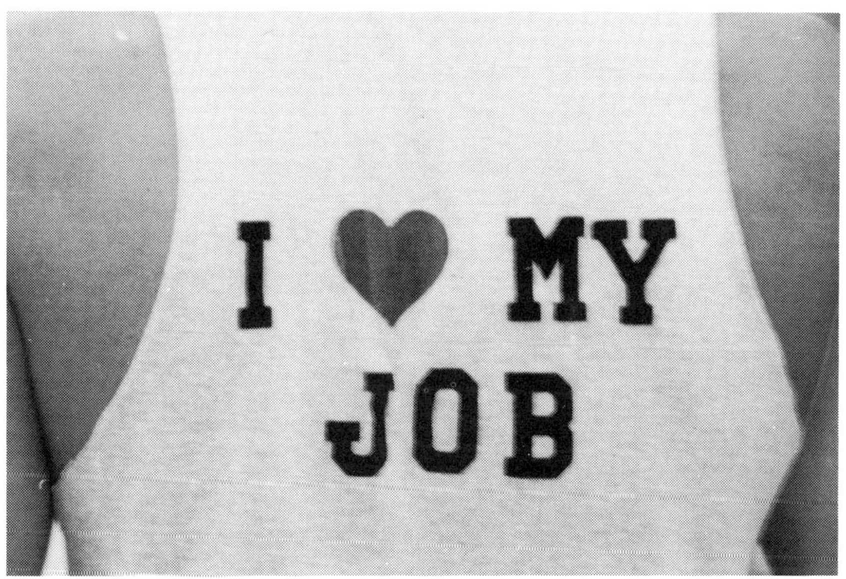

camp which ordinarily might not have been in their fields of endeavors. They learned things like the symptoms of a diabetic child, the life cycles of a turkey in the Texas Hill Country, and how to cure homesickness.

One counselor noted in an end-of-camp poem that he had experienced things that would never be forgotten, in addition to having one of the best times of his life. He wrote that his eyes had been opened to the true beauty that lies inside of others and himself. "I didn't know that I could give so much or receive so much. People become so close in such a short time, and what a blessing."

What did these counselors look like? They were all adult young people, some short and some tall, some blonde and some brunette. They walked; they talked and laughed; they were just young folks who liked loud music and their own kind of dancing. They looked like ordinary young men and women. But that was on the outside. Inside each tanned and muscular body they were medical marvels: they had nothing inside but one big compassionate heart. There was something else, too. There was a strangeness behind their eyes which was almost hidden. All summer long these young people had seen wondrous things they would never forget.

They had seen almost impossible acts of courage and endurance. There was a look of pride and personal accomplishment in their eyes, too, for they had received gifts few possessed: they had discovered the secret of how to bring from a small, disabled body a brave attempt to achieve; they had learned to raise from a child's lonely heart a happy spirit and a desire to interact with others. They went home after a summer at the Lions camp knowing they had received as many inspired gifts from the children as they had given. One camper, who later returned as a counselor, explained this by saying, "I just want to give back what you guys gave me."

Counselors at the Lions Camp spent fifty-six hours in pre-camp training and 1,440 hours on duty, with 240 hours free time. They were paid $100 a week for ten weeks to be a substitute mother/father, serve as big brother or big sister, be a friend, serve as a teacher of varied subjects, share secrets, provide a shoulder to cry on, give advice and love, serve as negotiator in squabbles, supervise good eating and health practices, pinch-hit for a counselor out on emergency, answer thousands of questions and sometimes the same one many times, be patient and understanding, pat heads and hold hands, be always fun and imaginative, keep kids busy, inspire camp pride, instill the 'I *can* do' spirit, be always on best behavior because a counselor will most of all be a role model to a lot of children who have been looking for one all of their lives.

It was not easy being a counselor on the job twenty-four hours a day; they slept with one eye open, a job not mentioned in the application booklet. Counselor applicants were very closely screened by the program department at the camp. This office received 175 to 200 applications from prospective counselors, out of which about 120 were picked.

An article in the *Kerrville Daily Times* written by Phil MacKaron had the following to say:

> An indicator of the camp's effectiveness is found in the counseling staff. Many of the counselors have physical handicaps and have attended the camp. A loose count showed one year that ten were deaf, four had cerebral palsy, two were visually impaired and some had missing or partial limbs.

The article went on to explain that a counselor-in-training, CIT, program was established for older campers who could not attend because they had reached age seventeen, but who wanted to be part of the effective and loving program.

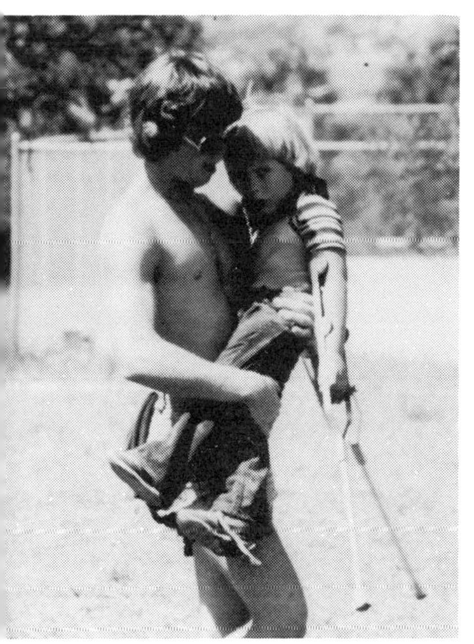
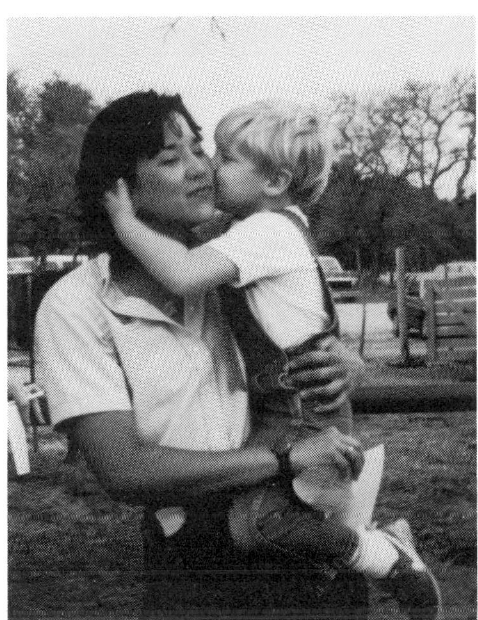

There was a special love between counselors and their charges.

Candy, age seventeen, had been at the camp since she was seven years old. Her right hand was missing at birth; but by the time she could be a CIT, she had no hang-ups. A leader in her school, she was an "A" student and a member of the National Honor Society. She commented on the lifelong friends a camper made at the Lions facility. As a CIT, she and others learned everything that was taught at the camp, working with each counselor. After becoming adequately trained, they could be hired as a counselor. Candy saw her role as a counselor as one of letting the kids have a good time and treating them like just a normal kid. "We don't try to hide the handicaps; we just teach them how to function with them, and ignore them." Director Glenn Crawford saw Candy a few years after she did not return to camp because of college work. She had graduated with a degree in recreation therapy and was ready to go out into the world and help others.

One summer a counselor in a wheelchair assigned a camper with a hearing disability to push him, then he instructed a vision-impaired camper to hold to the pusher and a mute to hold the hand of the second person. Finally that counselor's whole unit had formed a chain. The counselor said he didn't need that push. This was his way of keeping all his kids together.

Supervisor Lopez did his major recruiting of counselors in February each year, after having spent all winter organizing camp for the coming summer season. To obtain the best possible personnel, Lopez recruited at colleges and universities in Texas, Oklahoma, Arkansas, and Louisiana. "It's like a job fair," he explained. Students interested came to his campus presentation and received application forms. However, one of the major methods for recruiting counselors was by word-of-mouth, especially from the mouths of those enthusiastic staffers of other summers.

A counselor was not required to be majoring in such fields as physical therapy, occupational therapy, education, special education, medicine, recreation, or therapeutic recreation. However, if one of these degree goals appeared on an application, Lopez looked carefully at that prospective counselor. Many counselors had been in such fields of study as forestry, animal husbandry, psychology, journalism, and music. One of the happiest by-products of the camp were those counselors who came, learned, helped, and felt, then in the fall changed their major courses of study at college to special education or other fields closely associated with handicapped children.

Lopez believed that most of the counselors at the Lions camp made "better citizens tomorrow and better parents one day in the future."

Nurses at camp were the staffers who really "felt the pulse of the boys and girls," said Crawford. The kids came to them to complain, and then shared their secrets with them. Registered nurses were on 24-hour shifts in an eight-bed infirmary, busily taking care of tummy aches, skinned toes, and other minor needs. In emergencies, doctors were at the nearby Kerrville hospital on call. There was one nurse for the entire first summer of camp in 1953; in 1988 there were eight on duty.

The week preceding opening of camp every June, counselors attended a mandatory in-service training seminar given by Lopez and Program Director Rand Southard, permanent staff members, and a few outside lecturers. The camp's philosophy was "training and development of staff are essential to the delivery of quality care to the special children who attend Lions camp. The staff must be able to challenge the spirit of these children while maintaining a safe, non-threatening environment. It is the belief of the Lions League that each camper must be given the opportunity to develop to his fullest potential." The counselors were given every opportunity in their jobs for personal growth, development of professional skills and positive attitudes, and for experience in teamwork.

Classes during staff training began early in the mornings and ended several hours after supper breaks. They covered every possible area, from how to get a camper to relax in the swimming pool to duties at check-in times. Different classes were held for what the camp called the "Old Warriors" who were the returning counselors and the "Young Braves" who were new.

Some of the subjects addressed in training sessions included policies and procedures for the camp in general, daily schedules, counselor-in-training program, sign language, operations in the camp setting and on camp outs, parents' perspectives, children with hearing and vision impairments, recreation planning, review of child abuse, behavior management, how to plan and manage games and mixers, emergency procedures in all situations, risk management, group dynamics, goal-setting for counselors and campers, and wellness. Counselors learned to use emergency radios, proper flag ceremonies, how to handle the camp phone system, techniques for lifting and transfer of children, workings of orthopedic appliances, what to do with problems involving epilepsy, and how to monitor bowel and bladder functioning.

In addition, each counselor passed swimming, CPR, and first aid tests; then went through every activity a camper might experience, from canoeing and snorkeling to hiking and singing. To top it off, counselors were briefed on the last two weeks of camp which were devoted to children with diabetes. They acquired a general knowledge of this disease and learned how to handle special problems surrounding it.

Camp officials believed that no other element had greater therapeutic impact on a camper than did the interpersonal relationship between the counselor/instructor and the child. They stated that a person without a well developed sense of humor would not survive at a camp for exceptional children. Mistakes and funny incidents occurred daily, and the counselor who could not laugh would certainly cry. The counselor must have been able to laugh at himself and with the children.

At this special camp counselors needed the ability to be flexi-

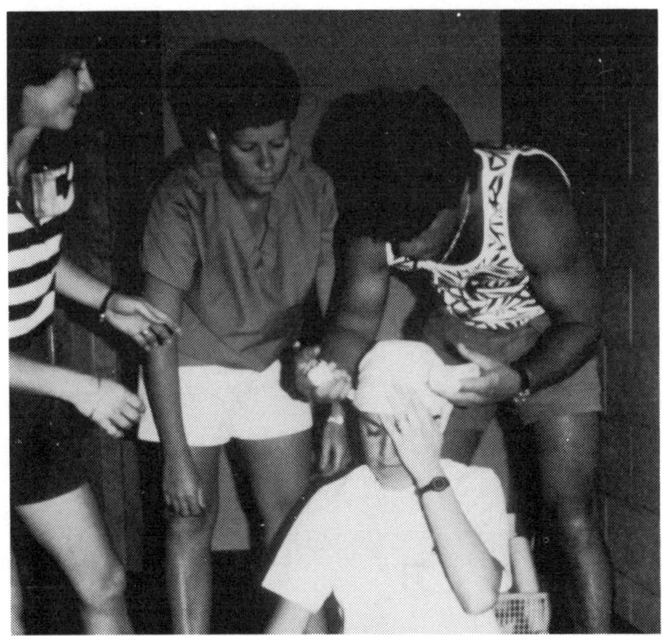

Counselors were trained in all activities, first aid, and coping with emotional problems.

ble, to understand the behavior of children, and to possess a certain degree of introspection and self confidence. A counselor must have been willing to learn, love children and exhibit acceptance of the children and of himself as persons.

Counselors heard the history of the Lions League camp and of Lionism in general, and they received constant evaluation by the program staff. During the pre-camp instructional session, the counselors read manuals written by staffers especially for the Lions camp, including the Staff Policy Manual of 140 pages, Counselor Staff Manual of 116 pages, Sign (language) Manual of 126 pages, Risk Management Manual of 100 pages, Nurse Policy Manual of 75 pages, Diabetic Manual, and Activity Plans for Summer Camp Manual.

Lopez was responsible for all counselor training. During summer seasons, he closely monitored them and assisted them with advice or help when needed. He gave them tips discovered by experience. Children ages eight, nine, and ten years were best to motivate because there was not as much peer pressure in that age group. On the other hand, older campers, fourteen through sixteen years, were sometimes easier to handle when they received little privileges, like staying up thirty minutes later and talking in the bunkhouse or they were given certain goals as definite challenges.

Homesickness came at almost any age. The first night or two were the hardest. Best thing, advised Lopez, was to keep them busy beginning with the very first day which was check-in time. On this day counselors had to work hard and really let their enthusiasm show. Sometimes when a camper cried from homesickness, a staff member urged them to write a letter home which represented a contact with the loved ones. Another effective method was to appoint the homesick child as a leader, immediately requiring his attention. Sometimes homesickness could be eliminated simply by asking that child to help the counselor.

Counselors did not allow the words, "I can't." A top goal of the camp was to take something negative and turn it into a positive thing. Counselors told campers in their wings that they could not roll over in bed and say, "I don't want to get up" like they did at home. The sun was up, so counselors and campers got up for a full day of work and play. Good relationships between wing counselors and the campers in their groups was most important in helping campers to develop positive attitudes and good skills at the camp. The wing counselors accompanied their children to every activity during the day, assisting instructors and keeping careful watch over their charges. There was one counselor to every three children.

Campers did not realize it, but most of their moves were monitored on a daily basis. Wing counselors and activity counselors made notes on each child, and communication lines were kept open between the activity instructors and the wing counselors. A lineup on behavior of a camper was noted on the first day of camp at check-in when a behavior coordinator held a brief conference with each camper. Among questions asked was "How do you feel about coming to camp?"

On the check-in day all counselors wore traditional khaki shorts and navy polo shirts with the Lions camp insignia. At times like this when the staffers met parents and Lion members from over the state, they became public relations arms for the camp. A mother commented on the staff, saying "I was so impressed with the way the counselors got along with all the children, just like one

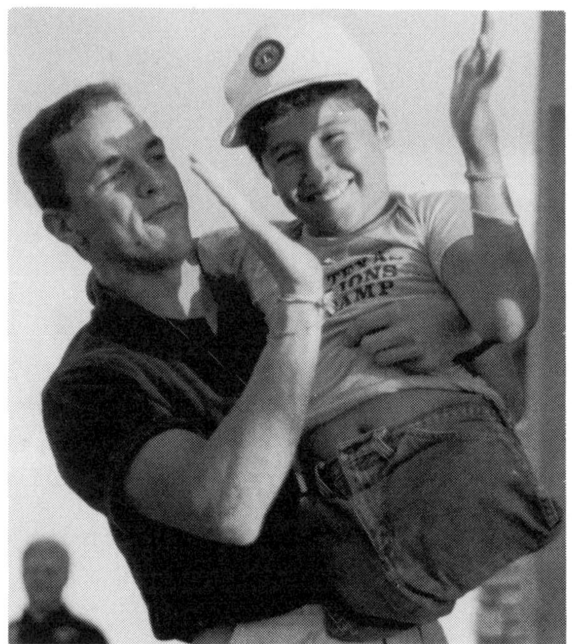

Counselor and happy camper.

big happy family. They cared, and there seemed to be so much love they felt for each other, too."

The young staffers generated camp spirit from the first night when they taught the new campers the camp song. The tune was borrowed from "Auld Lang Syne," and the words were:

> We're here for fun right from the start,
> so drop your dignity.
> Just laugh and sing with all your heart
> and show your loyalty.
> May all your troubles be forgot;
> let this camp be the best.
> Join in the songs we sing tonight;
> be happy with the rest.

Parents were pleased to learn that many of the counselors were former camp kids themselves. They could not help but feel a little more secure in the knowledge that these young people would really understand their special children.

Lopez said that some of the young college students came in wondering what life was all about; and at the end of a summer at the Lions camp, they realized that life was all about helping others. These counselors discovered, among all the hour-by-hour demands on their time, that they *could* give attention to everyone no matter what the needs. They also found that, like any other kid, at times they could really try a person's patience.

Said one counselor, trying to get a camper to make his bed: "What do you mean you can't do it? There are no 'can'ts' here. Find a way. I don't care if you don't have but one arm. Find a way!" One boy, who had been born without anything below his waist, insisted on a top bunk. He used his powerful arms and torso to scurry up the ladder to his bed in a hurry; he also could make his bed neatly. Campers with small hands that trembled had to labor long in the arts and crafts classes which were tedious. Counselors stood by urging them to try, try, and try again while suggesting ways to do the task differently. Statistics at the camp showed that next to swimming, kids like horseback riding best, with arts and crafts coming in for third in camper interest. Lopez said he thought they liked arts and crafts because they made something tangible which they could take home to their parents or friends; it was a visual success sign for them.

Times came when a counselor would need to carry a child to chase her first butterfly, but they did it gladly. Counselors spent lots of minutes urging a child in the pool to stretch an arm or a leg, pulling against the water to bring therapeutic grace to the body movements. A counselor might have to sit for an hour with a camper holding a fishing pole for the first time. This hour could be the time when peace entered a child's heart and brought him hope.

One mother reported that her child cried the first night back home because she missed camp and her counselor so much. When counselors picked children to receive certificates on Awards Night, they did not consider the fact the child might have achieved top rating in the activity. What was more important was how well he cooperated, how much he improved, how hard he tried. Every step completed in an activity by a Lions camper was a big accomplishment, and counselors shared the victories.

"My biggest problem" admitted a counselor of several years, "is getting too attached to the children. I may find myself saying 'why did this one have to be this way?' but, on the other hand, we mostly don't even think of them as handicapped at all. We think of them as just kids." When it was time for lights to be out one eve-

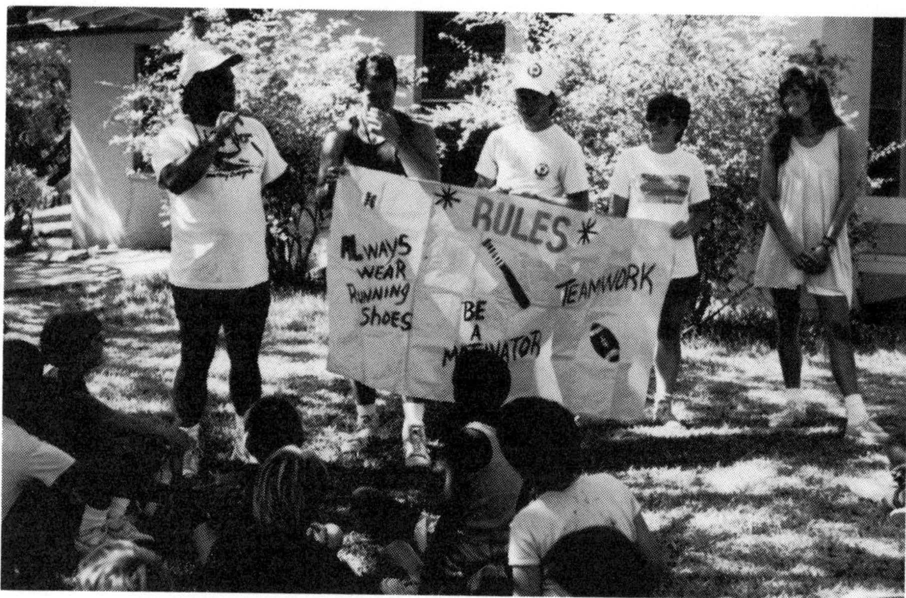

Safety rules were first things taught in any activity.

ning at camp and the children were climbing into bed, a wing counselor heard a tired kid say softly, "Thank you, God, for my handicap." Counselors got little notes all during camp, and then at their homes, that said "I love you."

Days for the counselors began before the children awoke and ended after they fell asleep. No matter what time it was, these staffers kept their spirits high and strictly followed their motto: "Drop your dignity." They clowned with the children and with each other. Everyone pinned a nickname on everyone else. The nature craft counselor might be "the snake lady," and there was always a "Tex." Wing counselors usually become the father/mother figure for the campers, but all counselors were special to the kids. To be one was the dream of most of the children. There have been some unusual counselors, like Terry Sylestine, a full-blooded Alabama-Coushatta Indian, who taught crafts and entertained with tribal dances, wearing full costume.

The eighty-two-year-old Eddie Martin wore many hats at camp. She drove for the mail each day, picked up children at the airport, took visitors on camp tours and was a top public relations person. A former Clifton, Texas, physical education teacher, Eddie called herself the "go-fer" of the camp. When she was with the Clifton schools she also drove a school bus and taught driver's ed. Thirty-two years ago, she began as the camp nature studies counselor. When Eddie was fifty-nine years old, she decided to enroll in judo classes; she won a "superior" rating.

Eddie was a historical storehouse for the Lions camp. She remembered a terrible storm came one night to disrupt an overnight camp out. She was herding five little girls with impaired vision to a waiting truck in the middle of the night. They were huddled under a blanket and shuffling along when one said, "Eddie, if I come back to camp next summer will you remember me?" Once Eddie selected a child to lead the Pledge of Allegiance at the morning flag-raising ceremony, and coached her about the service. The child got up on her wobbly little legs and yelled out, "Is this it, Eddie: my country tis of thee?"

A camper explained the Lions camp to a friend. "It's a place where you're happy no matter what kind of handicap you have! If you're blind, the counselors help you see. If you're deaf they help you hear. If you're crippled they help you walk. It's where you don't feel sorry for yourself any more."

Concluding counselor activities each summer was a staff banquet where the camp gave a boy and a girl counselor the Koennecke Scholarship Award of $500 each, provided the counselor used it for college. Recipients were evaluated on his or her service to the camp, and were selected by vote of all counselors. Also given was a Devotion to Youth Award to the outstanding male and female counselor selected by the staff. Similar to the Best Camper Awards, these were the highest honors counselors could receive.

It was necessary for counselors to joke among themselves; it was necessary that they had a little free time when they could have fun together. Romances bloomed among counselors every summer; some ended in marriage. At the end of camp, the counselors produced a newsletter to be read by themselves alone because it was very gossipy with "nothing sacred." It was called "The Summer That Was." Items like the following were printed:

> This was the summer of ants, chicken pot pie, fires in Unit 1, ants, stewed zucchini, ants, K.P., sleeping late in Real, ants, diarrhea, and ants. Special commendations to Susan and Grace for riding red wagons down to the front gate, which is a long, curving

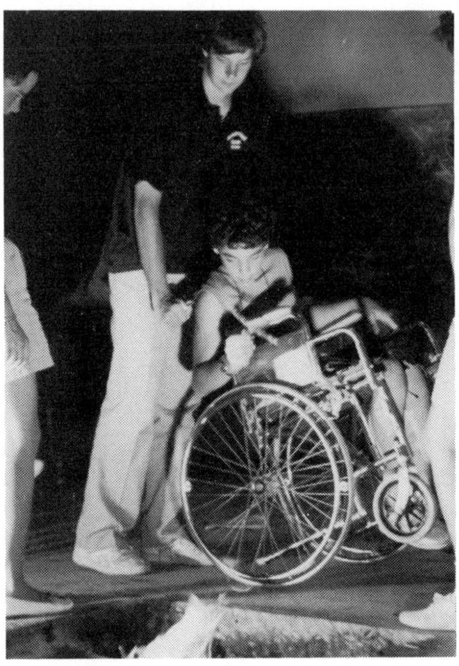

Counselor pushes boy in wheelchair to make his wish at traditional old Indian "stick ceremony."

road, but was topped only by Andy and Brian who rode wheelchairs down to the front gate. Among those exhibiting true Lions Camp Spirit in their actions were Tommy, who gave white paint instead of glue in Arts and Crafts, Greg who hitchhiked to the hospital with a camper who had a leg injury, Nancy who went to the Infirmary to get a lice shot, Celeste who wore a camper's shoes for three hours without knowing it.

The following "Beatitudes for Friends of the Handicapped" is from the *Catholic Standard* published in Washington, D.C.

> Blessed are you who take the time to listen to difficult speech, for you help me to know that if I persevere, I can be understood.
>
> Blessed are you who never bid me to "hurry up" or take my tasks and do them for me, for often I need time rather than help.
>
> Blessed are you who stand beside me as I enter new and untried ventures, for my failures will be outweighed by the times I surprise myself and you.
>
> Blessed are you who asked for my help, for my greatest need is to be needed.

Blessed are you who understand that it is difficult for me to put my thoughts into words.

Blessed are you who with a smile encouraged me to try once more.

Blessed are you who never remind me that today I asked the same question twice.

Blessed are you who respect me and love me as I am, just as I am, and not as you wish I were.

— Chapter 8 —

"Mother Nature's Classroom."

"You can't bring the outdoors into the classroom, so we take the classroom to the outdoors."

— *Chris O'Quinn, Program Supervisor, Outdoor Education Center, Texas Lions Camp*

There were six children sitting in a circle, passing around a crinkly snake skin. Each one felt it carefully, almost inch by inch, while the teacher explained the details of a snake's necessity for periodically shedding its skin. Next item passed was a fossil, followed by a live baby ribbon snake, a wild turkey feather, wiggly white rats and brown gerbils, and an assortment of leaves. None of the blind children were afraid or squeamish about the objects; each was eager to know the feel of animal life and the outdoors.

After this session in the little log cabin at the Lions camp, the children, the teachers in the Outdoor Education Center and the blind children's sponsors, hiked down an obstacle-free nature path, stopping along the way to feel the different kinds of trees and shrubs. They hiked to the pond, fished and studied different kinds of aquatic life, and listened to a tape on the sounds of the woods at

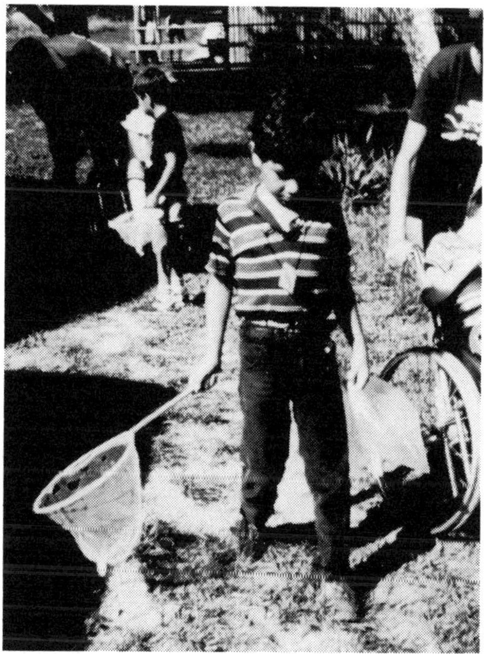

On a bug-and-butterfly hunt in outdoor education.

night. They sat still and listened to the real sounds about them, then talked about what they had heard. They enjoyed the warmth of the nearby campfire. They only expressed fear of the darkness and the fire, which teachers calmed with reassuring explanations of each situation. An outdoor education intern at the camp was surprised at their fear of the dark. Were they not always in the dark? Her supervisor explained that the children's mental sensory perceptions enabled them to realize "darkness" the same as a sighted child. The beliefs of children with or without sight can be similar. The opposite of vision is not darkness, just as the opposite of light is not blindness. One can perceive with the mind.

When the group returned to the bunkhouse at the camp to sleep, one eight-year-old boy insisted on sleeping on the top bunk. His sponsor did not say, "no," but did explain the safety risks. Although it would be the first time he had ever slept on a top bunk, it intrigued him and he was determined. The little fellow won a battle that night which gave him new courage and independence, as well as new knowledge of how this living skill was accomplished. Next morning after breakfast, the children were out on the grass and in

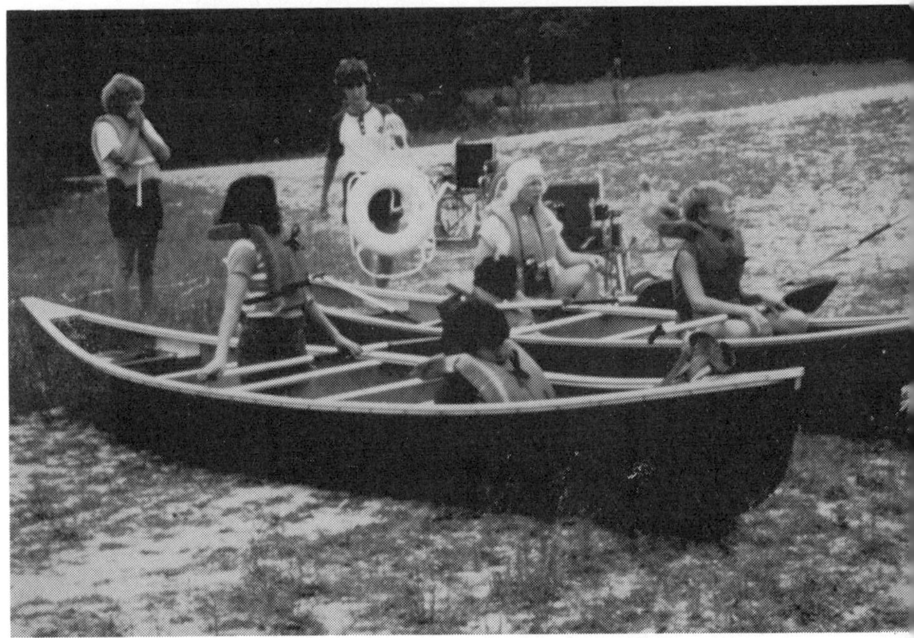

Children learned canoeing first on the grass.

the canoes placed there. They learned the feel of a paddle, how to use it, safety rules of canoeing and facts about water-traveling before entering the water.

Sometimes groups of children came during after-school hours for certain classes in this Texas Lions Camp for Outdoor Education. Other times independent school districts sent classes for a week full of lessons offered. The center was the only camp in the state which had been certified by the Texas Education Agency as an accredited private school. A key factor in obtaining this accreditation was the quality of the staff. Outdoor Education opened at the facility in 1984, with Gary Caves as the first director. He remained for two years, and effectively laid the groundwork for organization and operation of the services.

When the League discontinued its nine-month program for the blind, which had been in operation some twenty-five years, Director Glenn Crawford believed the new outdoor education program could be handled profitably and well at the camp, and the directors agreed. The concept originated in Houston at Camp Olympia where all of the hundreds of fifth grade children in the public school system were scheduled for trips to the camp every year.

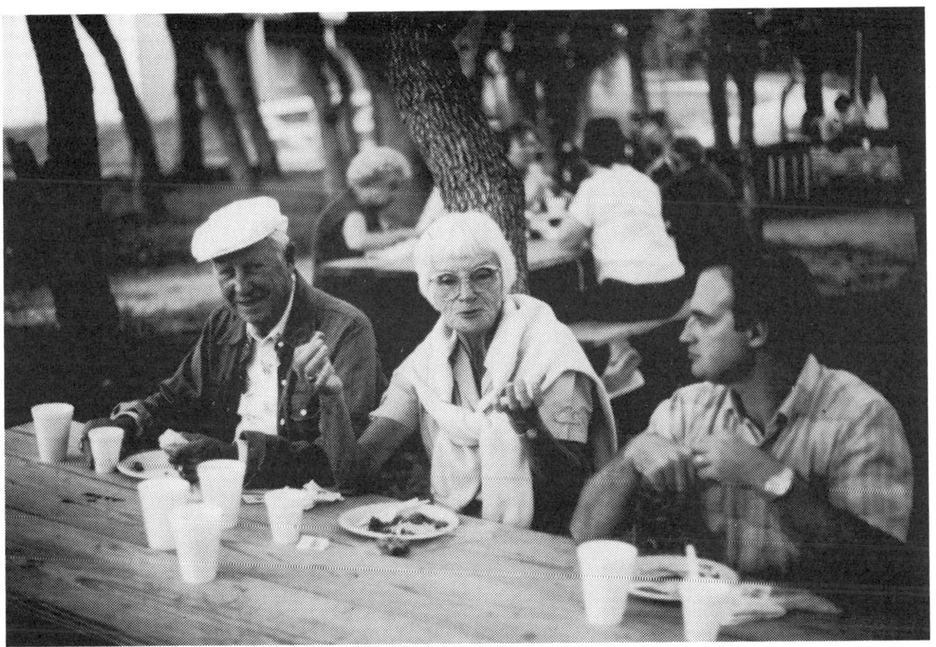

Senior citizens in Elderhostel program on cookout.

Originators called it a better way to learn, by experiencing sciences, even math and social studies, in an outdoor setting where there were hands-on teaching methods.

The Lions camp was uniquely equipped to handle all types of students because it had been designed for the handicapped, and the staff was trained in mobility techniques and sign language. Because of this, it drew a wide range of students and groups. The site and facility were gifts from Lions and caring friends who began the handicapped camping program in 1949. The outdoor education center was set up as a service for promoting physical and intellectual growth on over 500 acres of fields, woodlands, gardens and greenhouse, exercise and nature trails, horse stables, game fields and courts, conference halls, dormitories and dining hall.

The outdoor center was where a child would sit outside and learn. Courses were taken from the classroom and taught in the outdoors. Summer camp programs for handicapped children were estimated to reach only about one percent of the eligible children in the state. The Outdoor Education Program served a much larger percentage of these children, in addition to many without disabilities. The summer camp was free of charge; but the outdoor education program was supported by fees from the various schools, plus registration fees from other outdoor education programs held during the winter, such as Elderhostels, teacher workshops, group conferences and seminars, church retreats, private parties, and art shows. The Texas Lions Camp Education Center had professional workshops for teachers and parents, and among the groups who scheduled meetings there were the South Texas Regional Deaf Educators Conference, Texas Science Teachers Association, Project Wild Curriculums, National Conference of Lions Camps, Longhorn Recreation Lab, Texas Agricultural Extension, and 4-H Youth Programs. Money left after costs from this nine-months' activity, went into the summer Lions camp operations. Mike Lackey was the full time staffer in charge of bookings for the nine-month activity. His job was similar to leasing a hotel. Fees for the respective programs varied depending on what services the group chose and were based on a direct cost basis. Programs were designed to meet specific needs of individual schools or groups. Total programming included instruction, materials, equipment, administration, lodging, food service, on-duty nurse and overnight dormitory supervision.

One reason the Lions League decided to open the outdoor center was the belief that their facilities and resources should be used all year long to bring in funds, to help promote a type of learning which could not be secured any other place, and to stabilize their well trained staff members for permanent positions. In the camp's fortieth year, 1989, the program was growing; during the first year of operation 3,000 children came for outdoor learning, and the center and its staff began making significant advancements in leadership roles in the fields of rehabilitation and outdoor education.

When a group of deaf children spent the week at the outdoor center, they participated in a map and compass treasure hunt, studied the interdependency between animal and plant life, dug at a fossil excavating site, toured a taxidermy facility and heard a lecture by experts in biology. Wrote Victor Galloway, executive director of the Texas School for the Deaf: "This visit was an educationally unique experience for our students as well as teachers, who felt that this was an invaluable in-service training in the area of outdoor education. Our desire is to involve more students next year.

Thank you again for introducing this innovative alternative learning package of activities to our students."

Other areas covered by the outdoor center include wildlife adaptation, deer range management, soil conservation, wildlife habitats, cowboy lore, Spanish history of Texas, bird life, flint knapping, entomology, orienteering, native plants and dyes, and native American lore. No other camp in the world had an astronomy platform for searching the skies. The astronomy equipment was given to the camp by Lion Lou Ackerman of El Paso, who built such equipment as a hobby.

Outdoor Education Supervisor O'Quinn, who had a wide background in special and outdoor education, said reading about a snake or a leaf in the school room was just not like actually *feeling* it. "Imagine learning nutrition from a horse or history from exploring an Indian mound!" Learning math in the outdoors might seem strange, O'Quinn explained, but students could grasp math and be excited about it in such projects as measuring the volume of water in the camp pond. She thought the Lions camp's outdoor education program had unlimited possibilities and advanced to broader scopes.

One day a student attending an outdoor class after her regular school hours, came running to O'Quinn with the good news that the pretty little ribbon snake in the nature lab had given birth to twenty wiggly babies. In another class the students learned that there was a plant with a seed that looked like a helicopter, and another had a seed that looked like a screw. O'Quinn called them "designer seeds." Through the hands-on activities, students learned where seeds came from and conditions necessary for growing them. They compared the many seeds and plants in the camp greenhouse and along the nature trail, and children became "plant parents" with a take-home project. This kind of lesson was designed for preschool age and first grade children, said O'Quinn. On the schedule for the future was a complete, live barnyard. In lieu of live animals, the Barnyard Beasties class presented a multi-sensory approach to discovering characteristics of common domestic animals. In this class, camp outdoor education teachers utilized furs, feathers, bones, pictures, and sound tapes of barnyard animals.

Older children learned why an octopus could not live in a desert and why an armadillo could not live in a pond. This class was

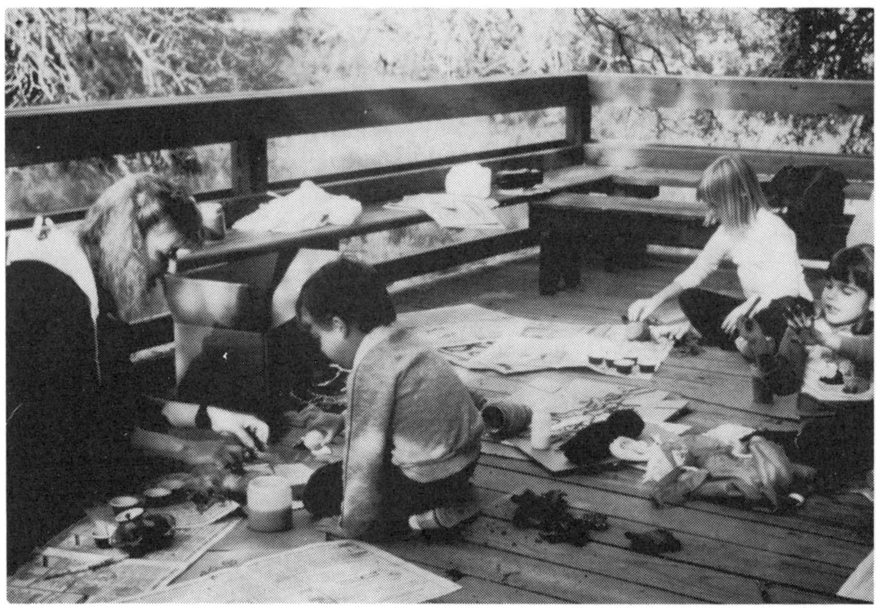

Outdoor lessons were always by hands-on technique.

entitled "Habitat Hopping." More advanced classes included studies of conservation, life sciences, primitive skills and outdoor survival. All classes provided the students credit at their schools; all were coordinated with the teacher and school district to satisfy grade level and curriculum requirements by the Texas Education Agency. O'Quinn employed interns for the school year who also received credit for their work at their respective colleges or universities.

The Lions outdoor instructors made all lessons fun. To learn about deer population management, a game was played in which students learned in the woods the grazing and foraging behavior of deer, their home ranges and food supplies, and survival statistics. In counting deer population and figuring future numbers, math was taught in connection with an exciting outdoor lesson.

One schoolteacher thought the rapport and "camaraderie" that developed between participants was one of the best things acquired at the Lions center. Another considered the most valuable "gift" her students received was the positive feelings they "got about themselves" where everyone was given the chance to be a winner in a cooperative effort. "It made me more willing to take the discovery approach with any kind of subject," commented a teacher who went through a course with her students. One said she found that while the students were learning, she was too. "We can grow together."

Crawford explained that the above attitudes were some of the main focuses of the innovative outdoor education at the Lions camp, as well as offering to all children, handicapped and non-handicapped, a chance to gain sensory awareness and understanding of the outdoors and its part in man's life. The atmosphere, he pointed out, was to encourage respect and cooperation among all environments through community living, group building activities, and group decision making. The teachers hoped that in addition to learning specific lessons and playing games, students would acquire extra-curriculum skills such as nutritional menu planning and conservation of electricity, paper and petroleum products.

O'Quinn brought her interesting experience to the Outdoor Education Center, having been involved in outreach programs, nature centers, parks and recreation departments, vocational training programs and child care projects. She was a graduate of The University of Texas and had studied in Guanajuato, Mexico.

At the camp, she headed other programs which were categorized under the Texas Lions Camp Education Center, including elderhosteling. Elderhostels were affiliated with the worldwide organization headquartered at Boston, Massachusetts. The Elderhostels were educational programs for older adults to expand their horizons and develop new interests. In Texas there were sixteen universities and five camps which hosted these senior citizens. The Lions camp offered three or more during the nine- months of fall-winter-spring. Most Elderhostels were one-week long and featured three specialized courses of one and a half hours each day. Many permanent staff members were involved besides O'Quinn, who also planned and supervised the activities outside the scheduled lessons, such as night parties and entertainments, cookouts, nature hikes, dancing lessons and archeology explorations. During some Elderhostels, Ron Anderson, director of development, lectured on early Texas history, treasure hunting, or fishing, as he was a nationally recognized authority on these subjects. Nolan Underwood, psychologist and public relations representative for the League,

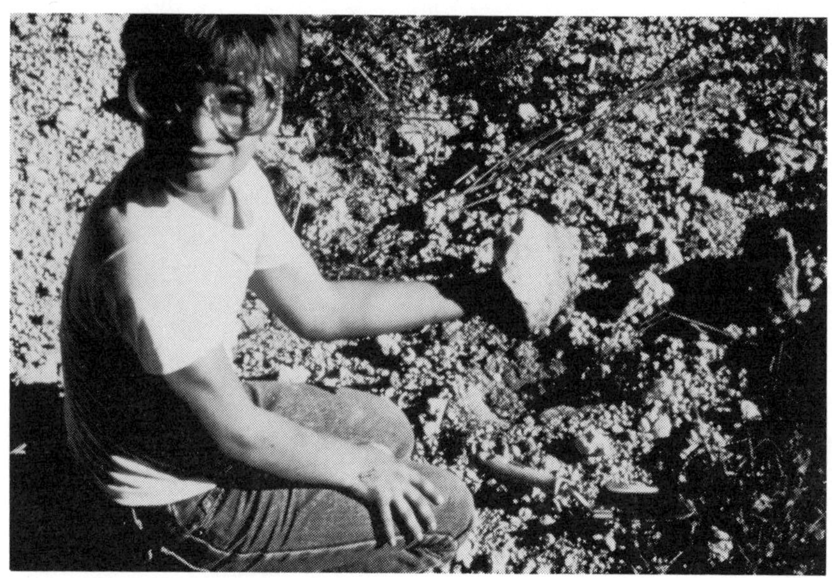

Successful "find" in archaeological diggings.

gave specialized programs on stress management and sensory perception.

During some of the Elderhostels at the Lions camp the senior citizens learned the art of making stained glass, learned all about the unique flora and fauna of the Texas Hill Country, and the history of famous Texas authors. O'Quinn made time during all elder programs for the guests to wander the trails of the camp, bird-watching or exploring nature; or to sit in a lodge and play dominoes and other table games.

Included in programs offered was the unique Family Learning Vacation, in which families attended with children who had the same or similar handicaps or chronic diseases. They all learned more about the handicaps, developed support networks and shared recreational activities. The exchange of ideas and information, plus the togetherness of fun, made this program another rehabilitative project for the Lions of Texas.

Crawford said he felt the Lions of the state considered all activities on their hilltop "mighty special." They were amply rewarded for their hard work, when they witnessed the delight of a blind child upon hearing the actual cry of a screech owl in the woods, having already felt the soft fuzz of some owl's feather at the outdoor center. The Lions knew they had accomplished their goal of service, he continued, when a hosteler's face turned into a smile upon digging up an arrowhead at the archaeological site. These were the people who had the opportunity of enjoying camp life at the Lions outdoor center.

Children who went to summer camp at the Lions facility were said to have left their handicaps at the gate. So it was with the people who came for outdoor education. The Lions offered peace and wonder, joy and love. Joann Cross, a girl who had cerebral palsy, wrote the following song while at camp:

> There's a light in my window that shines over me;
> and that light is a symbol that makes me smile;
> there's a bird in my window that makes me smile;
> there's a bird in my window that sings little tunes;
> and the air on my face smells like sweet perfume;
> the flowers that bloom are so pearly white;
> and the stars in the night are shiny and bright;
> forget all your troubles;
> they'll soon disappear;
> if you pray to the Lord,
> He'll always be there.

— Chapter 9 —

"Let This Horse Do My Walking"

"I saw a child who could only crawl,
mount a horse and sit up tall."
—from a poem by John Anthony Davis

It was rodeo time at the Lions camp, a brand new activity in 1988. The grand entry, with flags and music and riders all dressed up, had been concluded and the first contest of the day was the egg-in-spoon event.

Seven handicapped children mounted horses and formed a circle. Each had a spoon, in which a counselor placed an egg. This was a very delicate event, and contestants campers, counselor rodeo clowns and queens were quiet, for the first time. The riders spurred their horses, first walking, then trotting; the pace became faster and faster. Oops, an egg dropped, and that horseman was out of the race; then another one. The pace was fast now, two eggs dropped, and only three contestants remained. The crowd was yelling encouragement and cheering. The bumps took out another camper; two were left. Faster and faster went the horses in the cir-

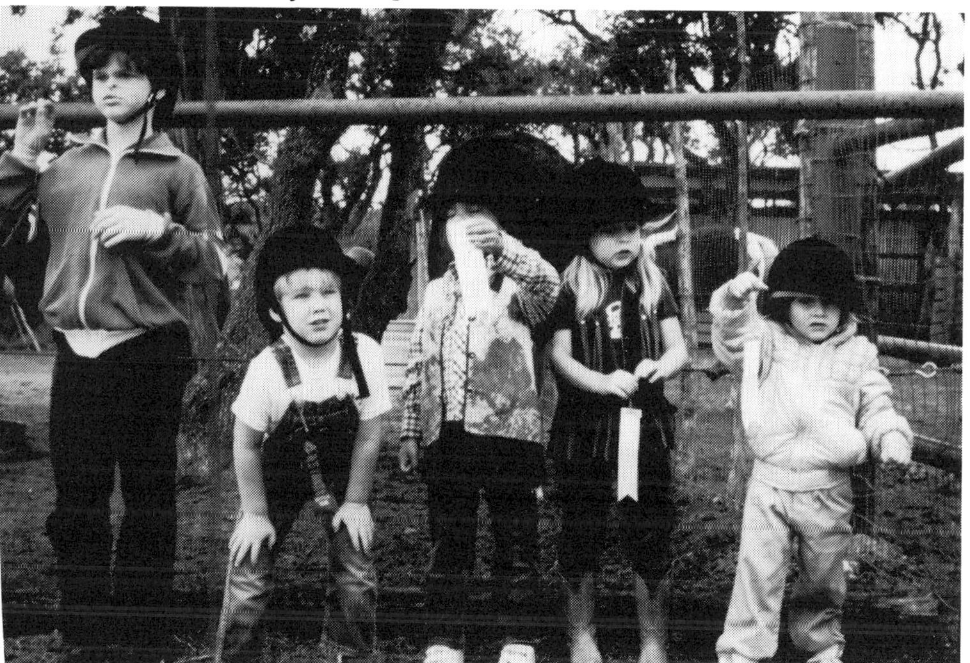

They were never too young for therapeutic horseback riding.

cle, until one dropped her egg while making a turn, and George was the winner!

Horseback riding proved to be a success that summer at the Texas Lions Camp, assuring the League that they could now go forward with plans to offer therapeutic riding lessons all year long as their newest help for the handicapped. Since summer camp did not accept emotionally disturbed children, the winter program would take in adults and the emotionally disturbed.

Keith Smith, supervisor of therapeutic horseback riding at the camp, pointed out that emotionally impaired individuals could benefit from horseback riding; blind persons also did well in therapeutic riding. Classes at the Lions camp complimented clinical physical therapy.

Therapeutic riding had its beginning in the ancient Greek culture where it was used as therapy for wounded soldiers. Since then, it expanded into Europe where it was widely used, and made its entrance in the United States in 1968. Since that time, the concept as therapy for many types of disabilities spread over the nation and became one of the newest trends in rehabilitative exercises.

The camp used horseback riding to help those having cerebral palsy and spina bifida, as well as amputees and children with vision and hearing impairments, said Smith. Horseback riding ranked second in popularity with all campers, being topped only by swimming. The barns, riding fields, and the huge modern arena were located on a hill that overlooked a panorama of valleys and lower hills. It was a place where a horseback rider could have felt very free and inspired. The Lions Club in the small North Texas town of Santo, which was chartered in 1985, bought some $10,000 worth of equipment, hauled it to the camp and built the arena. Crawford, who made the charter address when the Santo Club was organized, said that when lights were installed at the arena, the League would rent it for rodeos and horse shows.

Smith, who held a B.S. degree from Louisiana Tech in equine and animal science, attended the Cheff Center in Augusta, Michigan, in the fall of 1988, where he was certified as an instructor for therapeutic riding. He received advanced certification in western horsemanship with the Camp Horsemanship Association and was a member of the North American Handicapped Riding Association. He joined the Lions camp staff in 1987.

The camp owned twenty-one horses in 1988, and the campers wanted to make pets of all of them. Two of them were small, one of which was a Welsh pony. Big Mack, a black Tennessee Walker which Crawford drove to Tennessee to pick up, followed everyone around nuzzling for attention. Mack was not as bad about attention as Problem Solver, a one-time racehorse who had injured his knees. His owner, a young woman, gave him to the camp because she was dying of leukemia and wanted to make sure Problem Solver had a place to live where people would love him. Crawford said the big horse stuck a jagged tree limb through a part of his shoulder; and while he treated the wound three times a day, Problem Solver put his head on Crawford's shoulder and went to sleep.

Horses ridden in the program received regular training and were accustomed to wheelchairs, walkers, and unusual behavior. Special equipment at the horseback riding center included a mounting ramp to accommodate wheelchairs, hard hats, belts, and handholds for physical support, Devonshire boots and modified riding equipment.

Smith did not allow more than five horses and riders in the working pens or arena at one time for safety reasons. Most camp-

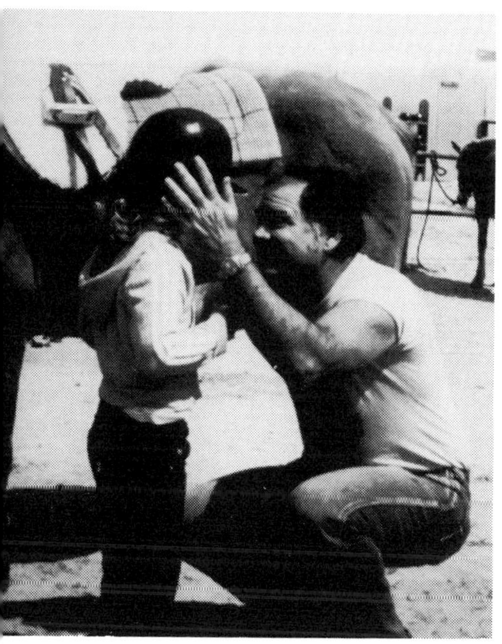

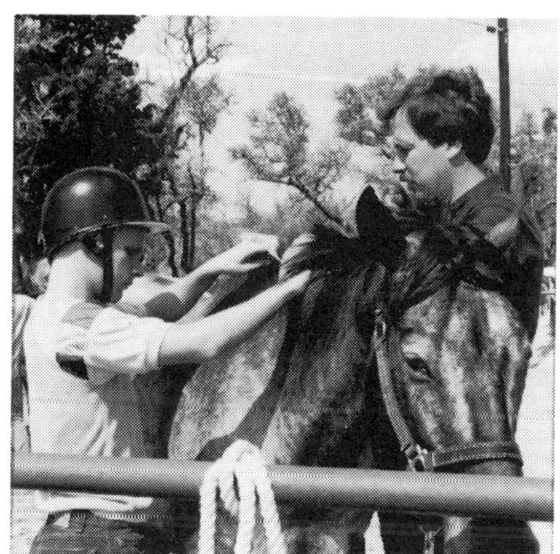

Daddy helped young horseback riding student with safety helmet, left. Student with vision disability learned all about a horse.

ers, as well as many in the winter horse program, were accompanied by one or two "side-walkers." These were volunteers or counselors who walked, or ran, beside the horse and rider to assure complete safety for the student. Summer campers rode for recreation, although therapy was a planned by-product. "We try to give them a skill they might be able to take back in their hometowns." said Smith.

Greg Holcomb, who assisted with the horses as a counselor, said one summer a small boy, with both legs in braces, came to camp from his ranch home. He did not want to ride horses, because he had tried many times on the ranch, but it always pained his legs. Greg took it very easy with him, urging him to just try for a minute. When it hurt, Greg asked him if he could stand it a bit longer until he got used to the position. In a few lessons with leg muscles stretched to normal flexibility, the boy was staying in the saddle as long as Greg would let him. His legs got use to the position, and he was so excited to think that now he could ride at the ranch with the cowboys.

Winter therapeutic classes brought money to the League; some students paid for the sessions personally, and some received scholarships donated for that special purpose. Since Lion members over the state placed confidence in community support for their camp operation, plans were formulating in 1989 whereby a community could sponsor needy persons who did not have funds. They were calling it Sponsor-A-Rider or Sponsor-A-Riding Session. Smith explained that charging for these lessons "allows us to break even with our horse fund while providing low cost therapy for children. In addition to utilizing the animals we have here we provide lasting therapy for the students." His definition of therapeutic riding was "actually working on a disability to try to reverse its effect, using the horse as the therapeutic tool." Remembering details of how to perform on a horse was used to build memory retention for learning disabled people, while it helped perception for the blind. Horseback riding could be very relaxing to persons who had cerebral palsy, and could help flex unused muscles. Smith explained that Downs Syndrome individuals were soothed by easy-gaited riding. For the physically handicapped, Smith picked a saddle that was best for comfort, either western or English. He estimated that at least ten percent of the general public were emotionally or physically handicapped. All of these could benefit greatly by therapeutic horseback riding.

Winter students at the Lions camp were from the Hill Country area, for the most part, and ranged in ages from three to eighteen, although it was not uncommon to see a senior citizen at the camp's Elderhostel program mount a horse and head for the hills. By 1989, the therapeutic horseback riding program at the Lions facility had become so popular that Smith received inquiries from San Antonio and Austin, and many were put on waiting lists. "We expect this outdoor program to keep growing," said Smith. "Right here in the heart of Texas ranching, there are many kids who have not been around horses." Smith planned to conclude each winter program with a horse show in mid-May that would be open to the public.

He offered lessons during the winter to children and adults who were not disabled, including western reining and show, English hunter, elementary dressage, and elementary and intermediate jumping. Like most of the programs at the Lions camp, horseback riding remained flexible, with lessons designed to fit individual needs. Smith felt that while classroom therapy was beneficial, a

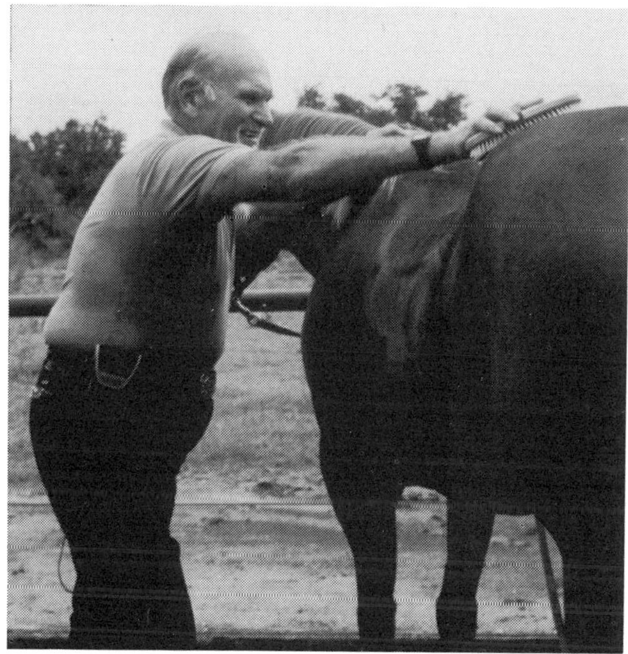

Blind adult began lessons by learning care of the horse.

change of pace would keep students' attention spans. "In riding therapy the students actually ride while listening to an instructor."

Students with missing legs felt good on a horse that was a sturdy base for them. They acquired a certain sense of independence, as well as balance. When riding a horse there was no need for crutches and wheelchairs. An added benefit was that the students themselves controlled the movements of the horse, which gave them new self-esteem. Smith said, "with self-esteem comes self-assurance; most of these students have never been off the ground, much less on a horse.

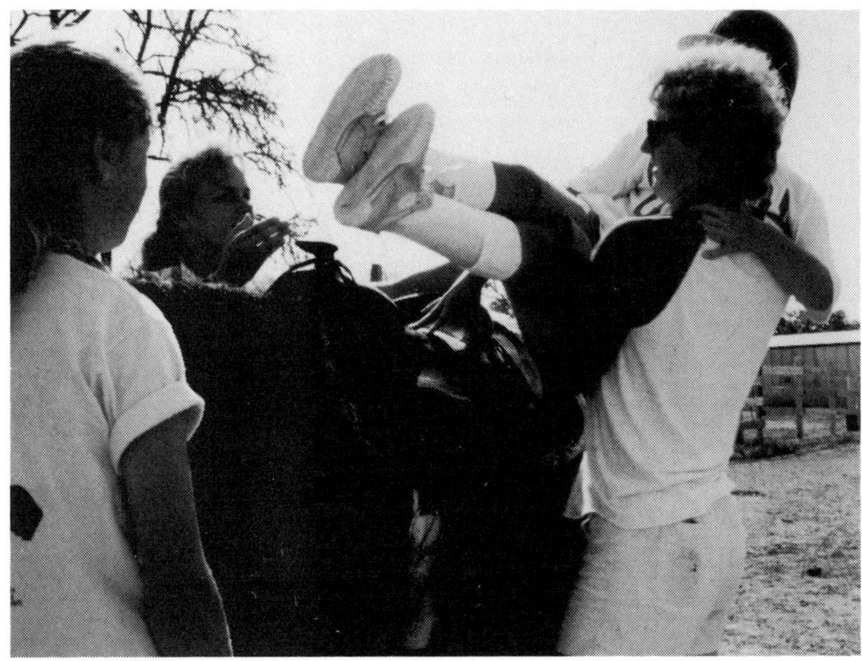

The horse could do the walking for their riders, who acquired confidence by learning how to control them.

What could take me
From the darkness of
My own powerlessness?
Can give me back
My pride?

See how boldly he prances
How he holds himself
As he dances,
His power and beauty
Move into me.

His whinney
Sings in my soul,
He uplifts me
Where I can meet
The world on equal terms.

His trust and affection
Are valuable rewards
I earn
By being responsive to his needs.
In giving care
I become worthy
Of receiving love.

His muzzle is velvet
Against my hand,
His eyes are full of
The esteem and magic
I wish to bring to
My life.
In respecting him
I share
His beauty.

— Lu Dudley 1987

— Chapter 10 —

"The Camp Tailtwisters"

"They are God's children, and all of God's children should have the same chance."

— Jack Wiech, First President
of the Lions League

Somebody had to do it. Somebody had to say, "No, we cannot afford that." Somebody had to yell, "Yes, we'll do it!"

This *Somebody* at the Texas Lions Camp was a combination of the governing board of directors and an executive director. That's the way the original bylaws of the camp were formulated in 1949. In Lions terminology *Somebody* was probably the closest to an official "tailtwister." Tailtwisting was peculiar to Lionism. A tailtwister was an elected official in every Lions club throughout the world whose job was to steer the weekly club meetings on an even course. He kept the business-at-hand moving, members on the subject and in good humor, and all discussions in line. Tailtwisters were supposed to handle their jobs in a lively, humorous, and knowledgeable manner.

One director/tailtwister said qualifications for his position were a strong back and a car with a big trunk. Directors carried the load for raising enough money to keep the camp operating, answering all questions about the camp, and keeping it constantly before the members of their respective districts. Since additional members meant additional camp funds, directors tried to keep Lions of Texas busy recruiting good new members. The director was the closest of any Lion to the camp and its activities, problems, and successes; he helped to make decisions for needs every year while planning for the future.

Directors were tailtwisters, and also the crucial liaison between the camp and the Texas Lions club members. It was necessary for them to not only think in business terms, but to think in terms of service to children, remembering the promise their counterparts made in 1949 to establish the best camp for as many handicapped children as possible. The directors were charged with keeping alive the camp spirit of *I can do* among the Lions of Texas.

Value of the nonprofit Texas Lions Camp, as estimated by Executive Director Glenn Crawford in 1989, was $15,000,000. With the operation in a big business category, the board members, executive committee members, and executive director and his staff were carefully selected. At the top of the Lions camp network in 1989 were the 40,000 Lions Club members throughout Texas who were the owners of the nonprofit Texas Lions Camp. It was their money and time that kept the camp alive, so they needed to have input into their investment at all times. This was done by electing the board of directors for the camp.

Included on the board, some eighty-two-members strong, were the elected governors of the sixteen Lion districts, all immediate past district governors, two Lions elected from each district, the executive committee, charter members of the board, and active past presidents of the League.

The Lions picked the board members; the board selected the executive committee; the executive committee hired the executive director, who was the full time top staff member accountable to the board. Officers of the executive committee included the president and immediate past president of the board; the first, second and third vice-presidents; the secretary, the treasurer, a representative of the state council of governors, and a representative of the elected directors. The network represented complete democracy in action and total Lions control.

Lifetime members of the board in 1989 included the only two

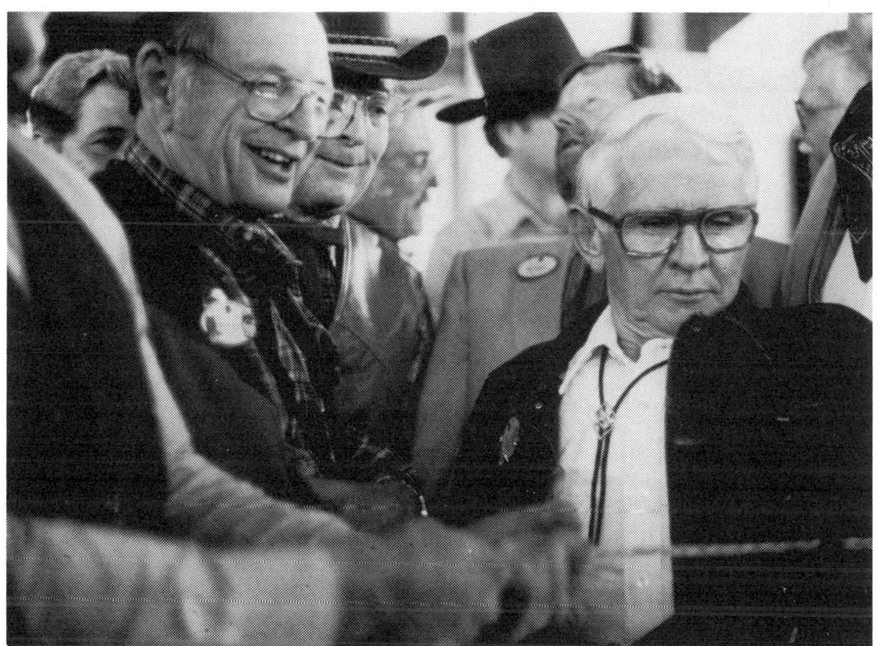

Lions loved to visit their camp. Here, from left are Jack Wise, a past district governor; Roy Davis, past president of the League; and Garvis Gilbert, first vice-president of the League in 1989.

living League founders, Jack Wiech and J. I. Moore; plus all past League presidents. Board members or any interested Lion could be appointed to one of the standing committees: bylaws, camp improvements, camp program, camper intake, diabetic program, finance, funds, security, and investments, historical, long range, membership development, planned giving and endowments, and public relations.

The Lion leaders who in 1949 founded the Texas Lions League, which was to organize a camp for crippled children, included W. R. Rutherford, Dumas; Schley Riley, Big Spring; Jack Wiech, Brownsville; Pat Jackson, Nacogdoches; Reagan Smith, Conroe; Virgil Minear, Hallettsville; and J. I. Moore, Kerrville. These prominent figures all were named as members of the first board of directors. They all signed the application for state incorporation of the camp as a nonprofit entity.

After incorporation of the League, Wiech was selected by the board as its first president. He guided the development of the ambitious dream for the next four years and saw it become a reality upon opening of the first camping season for crippled children in 1953.

Beginning with Wiech, every president was to meet the challenges almost daily of keeping the ambitious camp dream alive and moving. The following Lions have served as presidents of the board:

Frank Robertson, San Antonio, 1952–56
Reagan Smith, Conroe, 1956–60
Jim Ed Waller, Lubbock, 1960–65
Roland C. Jordan, Texas City, 1965–67
E. H. Munger, Houston, 1967–69
E. J. Grindstaff, Ballinger, 1969–71
J. P. McCracken, Cisco, 1971–73
J. L. McPherson, Houston, 1973–75
Sam Pakan, Shamrock, 1975–76
James Ward, San Antonio, 1976–77
Herbert F. Barsh, Waco, 1977–79
James H. Wheeler, Jr., Abilene, 1979–81
Fred Hamilton, Hockley, 1981–83
R. E. Price, Beaumont, 1983–84
Roy N. Davis, Weslaco, 1984–85
Raymond White, Hereford, 1985–86
J. L. Akridge, Georgetown, 1986–87
Marshall Cooper, Whiteface, 1987–88
F. Ray McLaughlin, Alpine, 1988–89.

One of the priorities for operating a camp as large and as successful as the Lions camp was selection of a strong and dedicated executive director. From 1949 to 1989, only three men served in this capacity. The first director was Frank Robertson, who guided the operation for twenty-three years; next full time director was J. L. McPherson, 1975 until 1978; Glenn Crawford took the reins in 1978 and was still director in 1989.

The dream of the Lions Camp for Crippled Children exceeded all expectations from the very start. By its fourth year of operation, 1956, it was already known among service organizations as "The Million Dollar Lions Club." It was the first statewide Lions project attempted in the nation. The founders and succeeding decision-makers set a solid background for obtaining necessary funds to run their Million Dollar Camp.

Supported solely by work and contributions of the Lions and

their friends, the League's bankroll was based on a unique dues-sharing plan approved by all Texas Lions clubs. This was an annual contribution of $12.00 from each member's dues to the camp. It was mandated by an amendment to the Lions state constitution.

Three types of memberships in the League brought in funds: anyone contributing $10 per year became an active member; persons contributing $25 were designated as sponsor members; and life members gave $100 or more per year. Life members received a certificate and a gold pin which was to be worn next to the heart. In addition, a club could secure designation as a "100% Participation Club" by contributing in any fiscal year a sum equal to $10 per capita of the total membership of that individual club. This became highly competitive between Texas clubs. One Lion said that if all the clubs in his district became 100% Participation Clubs, he would give an additional $10,000 to the camp. The Conroe Lions Club has been the only one to maintain its 100% Participation Club status throughout the entire history of the Lions League camp. Another enviable record was set in 1987–88 by the Rowlett Lions Club which reached an all-time high in 100% Participation history by collecting so much money per member that they reached an amazing 6700% Participating.

The Century Club was another funding group formed by the League under which donors gave from $100 to $5,000 in a single year. These supporters, some of whom were non-Lions, received a special lapel pin and a large, key-shaped plaque for their walls. Many Lions and their friends, as well as some organizations, remembered the children's camp in wills and memorials. A Book of Golden Deeds, which was kept at camp, listed every person who had a life membership.

Monies received from these sources went into four specialized funds: the general fund from dues, membership contributions, outside donations, and earned interest income, used for operation and maintenance of the camp; the endowment fund, from gifts, bequests, and contributions of money and property, which was kept separate from other League funds and of which only the earned income could be expended; the trust fund, from all testamentary gifts not designated for special purposes, which was kept separate, and of which only net revenue was used as determined by the board; and the building fund, administered by the executive committee, a depository annually of an amount equal to the depreciation of the total original cost of the fixed assets having been withdrawn from the general fund and kept separate to be used for replacing fixed assets when they were used up.

The accounting firm of W. L. Robinson in Kerrville was the accountant for the camp for about twenty years. Robinson was a Lion and contributed many hours of time and expertise, as well as his own money, toward the success of the camp. He set up the first general ledger, a tentative beginning operation budget, and the camp financial system. He served on the League's financial committee for thirty years. His wife, Effie, who worked with him in the business, was a Lioness and still active in 1989.

She remembered the early board meetings which lasted past midnight and into morning hours. "There were so many things to iron out in those days." In the camp's fortieth year, board meetings began at 6:45 A.M. Saturday, and it was usually 2:00 or 3:00 A.M. Sunday before the executive committee concluded its business. Mrs. Robinson said that first summer of camp operation, when the League had $250,000 on which to operate. "We spent every dime, so then we had to go back and get to work. We had learned that dues would not be enough."

Every director of the board had specific duties outlined in the Texas Lions Camp directors' booklet, and they followed them. The League believed in educating its representatives, so each year directors were asked to attend a special seminar at the camp where they received instructions on the League and its activities and where they also became campers for a day to see what it was like to camp at the Lions facility. Through the years, directors had taken their jobs very seriously. Some made it a full-time job. They remembered that they were the Texas tailtwisters and the keepers of the camp's flame of life.

Even in this area of the League's official domain, there was a provision in the rules for a "100% Director Award," because the League had left no stone unturned in trying to recognize all those people who worked so hard for the children. Mandatory for becoming a 100% director was to attend three League board meetings during his term, give thirty or more presentations to Lions Clubs or other groups during his two years, and attend at least one League orientation seminar during his term. In addition, a 100% director must have fulfilled at least three of the following: held at least one

League information booth at a district meeting, gave a camp presentation at a district convention, had half of his district clubs be 100% Participation or have a 10% annual increase in 100% Participation over the previous year, have camper participation every year, arranged a speech from a full time League employee at a district convention per year, or had an increase of twenty-five Century Club members during his two-year term.

Every director of the camp will put in numerous hours on paperwork, keeping the administrative office informed on his performance and successes. The executive director, in turn, kept each of the directors posted on the financial status of the camp and plans via a monthly report.

In 1989, Crawford said all the directors with whom he had worked for the previous twelve years had possessed a "vision to see and a courage to act," which Lions Founder Melvin Jones said all Lions must have. Crawford explained that the camp program went beyond its publicized goals of education and rehabilitation of handicapped children while giving them fun at camp. He said "We're really headed toward helping them to become responsible, employed citizens in adulthood. We like to feel we are helping to build America, and Lionism has always meant patriotism. We can't sit still when we are serving mankind; we must move up. I feel the Lions of Texas have every reason to be proud of the job they have done and are doing." Crawford pointed out that in 1989 fifty percent of the adult handicapped were unemployed on a national scale. Some were trained and educated, but did not have the opportunity to work.

At one director's seminar, men and women went to Inspiration Point to conclude the evening's activities. It was dark except for the big campfire which cast shadows on the faces of the people who were participating in a camp traditional wish stick ceremony. On this night, instead of young and eager faces, the fire flickered on adult faces wrinkled with feelings. These were the "tailtwisters" who had been entrusted with the duty of keeping alive the camp dream.

Each director stepped forward, blew a wish into a stick and threw it onto the fire. One said "Last week a diabetic girl we sent to camp came into my office to hug my neck. I am thinking tonight about the other five whose parents wouldn't let go. I promise to go back and work to get more of them to camp next summer." Another said he wished he would be able to get every club in his district to become 100% Participation. An older man admitted he thought he was about through with so much work in the Lions clubs after his term of directorship, but, now, he was going to keep trying for as many years as possible.

Each director made his wish, blew on his stick, threw it in the fire and let the smoke carry it up and over the hill country, in hopes the wish would be granted. It was an old Indian legend which the children loved. Then they all held hands in the traditional Friendship Circle, and concluded the campfire by singing the campers song. It was time to leave the meaningful scene. Inspiration Point had a way of "getting to you."

These were just tailtwisters like the many before them, going beyond the expected duties. They had assisted in transporting children to and from camp and had helped secure clothes and necessities for their children campers. They had been good promoters for the camp. When they visited the hilltop camp, they saw exactly what Texas Lionism was all about. During their terms most directors had spent a lot of time at summer camps, making friends with counselors and children; lending support and encouragement; and attending the emotion-packed Awards Night where their spirits, like those of the children, soared so high they felt they were almost to heaven.

LEAGUE DIRECTORS

Abbey, W. M.
Abella, Jess
Ackerman, Louis
Adams, Hal
Adickes, Leon
Adkins, Marvin
Akridge, J. L.
Alexander, Ralph
Alford, J. R.
Allen, Charles
Allen, J. Marvin
Alphin, D. H.
Anderson, Dexter
Anderson, Don
Anderson, Mark
Armstrong, A. J.
Arnold, R. M.
Ashlock, Ray
Ashton, Boyd
Atkins, D. L.
Atkins, E. L.
Atkins, Marvin E.
Atkinson, Jerry
Auvenshine, Bill
Ayub, Carlos
Backer, Donald
Baggett, Jack
Baggett, John
Bahnman, H. W.
Baker, Ben
Ball, William E.
Ball, William F.
Banks, Billy
Banks, Robert
Barajas, M. B.
Barrington, J. E.
Barsh, Herbert
Barsh, Robert F.
Bass, Robert
Bates, Byford
Beaird, Robert B.
Beakley, Penn
Bean, Claude E.
Beard, George M.
Beauchamp, Doug
Beauchamp, Harold
Beaver, Bill
Beck, Billy Bob
Beck Walt
Beckman, Roby
Bednarz, Tommy
Beggs, Ray
Belcher, Bert
Bell, James E.
Bell, Ronald
Bender, Fred
Bentenbough, Ron
Bigler, John
Binder, Robert
Blankenship, Lytle
Blase, Thomas
Blezinger, Clinton
Blume, Edwin
Boling, Ross
Boren, Richard G.
Borgfeld, Henry
Borman, James
Boswell, Carroll
Boswell, L. D.
Boulet, Wilbert
Bourland, Les
Bowers, Farley M.
Bowman, Fred
Boyd, Larry G.
Bozeman, Paul A.
Brabham, C. L.
Braddick, A. G.
Brancell, Harland
Brandon, Hiram
Brandt, B. L.
Bray, Cecil
Brenneke, Norwood
Bridges, Cecil
Briggs, C. P. III
Brinkman, A. H.
Brooks, Lester
Brown, Albert
Brown, F. Hall, Jr.
Brown, George
Brown, Hayden

Bruton, J. Harry
Bryson, Duane
Bryson, Gordon
Buckalew, Don
Buenger, Walter
Burge, John
Burnsed, Rogers
Burton, Felix
Burton, Jack
Busch, Emmett
Bushong, George
Butcher, Bill
Butler, M. P.
Caddell, M. N.
Caldwell, Allen
Caldwell, T. F., Jr.
Campbell, Louis
Campbell, Luren
Carmichael, Vernon
Carothers, L. D.
Carothers, M. E.
Carrillo, Thomas
Carrington, Jan
Carrington, Vern
Carroll, O. I.
Carruth, C. E.
Carter, Ellis
Carter, Roy
Cassle, Tim
Castellano, Ruben
Cathey, J. M., Jr.
Chadwell, Sidney
Chambliss, Roy
Chamness, Archie
Chaney, Don
Chapman, Lloyd
Chappell, Leslie C.
Cheaney, Theo
Cheatham, Roger
Cheek, T. Lovie
Cherry, J. H.
Cherry, Lynn
Childers, Joe
Childress, Hugh
Church, E. H.
Clare, John, Jr.
Clark, Tommy
Claxton, M. G.
Cocran, F. L.
Coffey, Robert
Coldeway, W. G., Jr.
Coleman, Walter H.
Combs, Don
Comisky, Ben, Jr.
Conner, George
Conner, H. E.
Connor, C. R.
Conrad, Frank
Cook, Art
Cook, James
Cook, Jim
Cook, Olden
Cook, Oscar
Cooley, C. R.
Cooley, Charles
Cooper, Cecil
Cooper, Eugene
Cooper, Marshall
Copeland, Kenneth
Coppedge, Rex
Corder, William H.
Cornelius, Leroy
Cornett, Leighton
Costa, Reynold
Cowan, Merle
Craig, Lee
Crane, K. T.
Crass, Clinton
Crawford, Clyde
Crawford, Guy W.
Crocker, Paul
Cross, Clinton
Cryer, Curtis
Cully, S. R.
Culver, Jim
Cummings, Joe Don
Curtin, James
Cutshall, C. C.
Daniel, H. B., Jr.
Dansby, Roland
Daugherty, Jas.L.
Davenport, Rodney
Davidson, Weldon
Davila, Fidel
Davis, Bob L.
Davis, C. E.
Davis, Oscar
Davis, Roy
Davis, Williams
Davlin, Stanley

De Wees, Darwin
DeVault, Gerald
DeVore, Russell
Dealey, W. A.
Delawder, J. A.
Dempsey, Jack
Dewberry, Maurice
Didlake, W. W.
Diebel, Burton
Dominguez, Fred
Donaldson, Oran T.
Dotson, Gordon
Downs, L. E.
Drain, Kenneth
Drever, Crawford
Dreyfuss, Harold
Duckworth, Earl
Dudley, George
Dyer, J. D., Jr.
Dyess, Lamar

Eads, John
Edlemon, W. L.
Edwards, Frank
Eiland, Paige
Eldelman, W. L.
Elledge, Bob
Elliott, E. H.
Elliott, Marshall
Elliott, Ray
Ellis, Bill
Ellis, David
Engels, Eugene
Estes, John W.
Evans, D. A.
Evans, Neil

Fain, Calvert
Fain, Calvin
Faubion, C. E.
Ferguson, Thomas
Ferrell, Edward
Field, Noble
Finley, Tom
Fisher, Billy
Fisher, Burt
Fisher, C. L., Jr.
Fisher, Joe J.
Fletcher, Howard, Jr.
Flood, Edwin
Flynn, Warren
Folk, Walter, Jr.
Fowler, John W.
Francis, Jasper
Francis, Thomas
Francis, Thocil
Franklin, Wallace
Freeman, Larry
Freeman, Nathan
Friedrich, H. L.
Fuller, L. K.
Furr, Sam
Futch, George, Jr.

Gann, Tom H.
Garcia, Wenceslao
Garett, H. R.
Garrett, Raymond A.
Garwood, Floyd
Gayle, J. Ray, Jr.
Geistmann, Clarence
Gentry, Fred
Gentry, Geo. P.
Gernentz, John, Jr.
Giametta, A. J.
Gibbs, John R.
Gibson, Allen
Gilbert, Garvis
Gilbert, P. J.
Gillette, Gordon
Gilligan, Neil, Jr.
Giroux, Roger
Glasin, John
Goetz, Joe
Goldfield, Max
Goldstein, Hirsch
Goldstucker, R.
Gonzales, Ben
Gonzales, Roger
Gooch, Larkin
Graham, C. Howard
Gray, Norman
Greene, Van
Greenfield, Larry
Gregg, E. R., Jr.
Gresham, Wendall
Grett, Cy
Griffin, Alton
Griffin, Fabrian
Griffith, Louis
Grindstaff, E. J. "Ebb"
Grounds, Jack
Gruby, Wm. J.

Guidry, Syd
Guinn, E. D.
Guither, Myron
Gullickson, Weldon
Haan, Robert
Hafley, Floyd
Hagler, J. W.
Hall, F. A.
Hall, Hulon
Hall, John
Halstead, Harley
Halter, Joe
Hamilton, Darrell
Hamilton, Donald
Hamilton, Fred
Hanson, Leonard
Harang, Paul
Harbin, J. H.
Hardin, George W.
Hargraves, C. L., Jr.
Harmon, Fred
Harrington, Howard
Harris, Jack
Harris, Joy C.
Harris, Orville
Harris, Thomas
Harris, W. C. O., Jr.
Harrison, Ardie
Hartwick, L. E.
Harvey, Dewayne
Harvey, Marshall
Harwell, Edward M.
Heard, Charles
Heath, Dan
Heath, Horace
Henke, Henry Joe, Jr.
Henry, Ralph L.
Herron, Loyd
Herschleder, Fred
Hicks, James
Hielscher, C. N.
Higdon, William
High, Ben
Hiler, Irvin
Hill, Homer
Hill, Olin
Hinkle, J. T.
Hodge, Homer
Hogge, William
Hollingsworth, Grady
Holm, H. O.
Hood, H. B.
Hord, Edwin
Horn, W. S., Jr.
Houston, J. A.
Howard, Benny
Howell, Duane
Howsley, Andy
Huchinson, I. R.
Huckabay, James
Hudson, Bill
Hufford, Leroy
Huffstutter, Bobby
Hughston, Ray
Hull, Robert
Hunt, Harold E.
Hunter, Wm. F.
Husencia, John
Huss, Russell
Hyde, Carl
Ingle, Harry
Ive, John J.
Jackson, Pat W.
James, Bill
James, Ken
James, Virgil
Jara, Al
Jesperson, Wes
Jeter, Steel
Jimerson, Duke
Johnson, Henry
Johnson, James R.
Johnson, Leonard
Johnson, P. E., Jr.
Johnson, Paul
Johnson, W. J.
Johnson, Wilbur
Johnston, Dr. Gary
Johnston, Perry
Johnston, Ray A.
Jones, W. M.
Jones, Calvin
Jones, Doran
Jones, George
Jones, Glenn
Jones, J. L.
Jones, J. T.
Jones, J. W.
Jones, Remus L.
Jones, W. E.

Jones, W. M.
Jordan, Jack
Jordan, Roland
Kahlich, David
Kahlich, Roy
Kallies, George
Karrer, Bert
Kaster, James J.
Kay, Marvin
Keas, Frank
Kelly, E. P.
Kelly, Frank
Kelton, A. W.
Kendrick, John
Kerstetter, Fred
Kimbler, D. O.
King, Charles
King, Ed
King, Wm. E.
Kirby, John
Kirndoll, Benny L.
Klein, Bernard
Kline, A. Lewis
Knight, Charles
Koenig, Don
Koennecke, Robert
Kolodize, William
Koonce, Robert
Kuykendall, C. F.
Labove, J. R.
Lacey, Hal
Lane, John
Larimer, O. V.
Lasater, M. H.
Laufer, Hyman
Laurie, Milton
Lawrence, Eldon
Lawson, Ben
Lee, "Rocky" Rex
Legendre, Paul H
Legg, Lonnie
Lemons, Jim
Lenzo, Joe
Leroux, Frank
Levertt, C. Howard
Levo, Bob
Lewallen, R.
Lewis, A. Lewis
Lewis, Raymond
Lewis, Teairl
Ligon, D. L.
Lindow, A. E.
Lindsey, Dr. Tom
Lindsey, Sam
Lipham, J. H.
Lipham, J. M.
Lipscomb, R. A.
Locke, John
Long, James
Longley, John
Love, Harold
Lucas, Henry
Luna, Francisco X.
Lundy, Robert
Luschar, Herman
Lyle, R. H.
Manchel, R. E.
Manley, R. M.
Manry, James
Maples, Loren
Marshall, James
Martin, J. T.
Martin, Roy
Martin, Sam
Martinez, Braulio
Martinez, Guadalupe
Maruska, Jerry
Massey, Cecil
Massey, Dale
Massey, Sammie
Mathena, Neil
Maudlin, W. D.
May, John A.
Mayberry, Paul
Mayer, Don
Mayer, E. B.
Mayers, Larry H.
Mayfield, Bill
McAdson, Lloyd
McAlexander, Walt
McAlpin, Willie
McAmis, J. D.
McBride, L. H.
McBryde, W. L.
McCain, C. E.
McCain, Carmen
McCollough, Jack
McCowan, C. A.
McCracken, J. P.
McCreless, G. S.

McCullough, Jack
McDonald, W. R.
McGann, Jack
McKusker, Carl J.
McLain, John
McLaughlin, F. Ray
McLeaish, Bob
McLean, J. E.
McLean, Julian
McLeod, Johnny
McMeans, Russell
McMinn, William
McMurtry, E. Hoyse
McNeill, James, IV
McNutt, Guy
McPherson, J. L.
McPherson, W. B.
McRae, H. L.
Meador, Boyd
Mehner, Philip
Meissner, Raymond
Melton, Bill
Meyer, Kurt
Keyer, W. E.
Meyers, Bill
Meyers, Larry H.
Miller, Jerry
Miller, T. L.
Miller, William
Millican, Ronnie
Mills, Fred
Minear, Roy A.
Minear, Virgil
Mitchell, David
Mogford, James
Mooney, Johnnie
Mooney, Johnny
Moore, J. I.
Moore, Roger
Moritz, Sylvan
Morris, Milton
Morris, T. D.
Morrison, Thomas
Moss, Mike
Muckleroy, Jimmie
Mueller, W. E.
Munger, E. H.
Musick, Elmer, Jr.
Myer, William E.
Myers, Felix
Myers, M. M.
Nail, Clyde R.
Naylor, J. W.
Neelley, Lloyd
Nelson, Jack
Nelson, W. T.
Neuman, Ed A.
Newman, James
Nichols, Raymond
Nichols, T. K.
Niemeyer, W. R.
Nipp, Tom
Nite, Marvin
Noble, M. E.
Noone, E. F., Jr.
Norwood, Charles
Nunley, Robert
O'Donnell, A. P.
O'Donnell, W. P.
Ochsner, Hal
Ortega, Homer
Osborn, J. D.
Owens, H. A.
Painter, John
Pakan, Sam
Palmer, Clarence
Palmer, Harvey
Palmer, John
Palmer, Paul
Parish, Joe
Parker, Bob
Parker, Williams
Parker, Wm. Preston
Parr, Joe
Parr, Paul
Partridge, Frank
Passmore, J. R.
Patrick, J. M.
Patton, Winston
Pavlik, Stanley
Payne, W. M.
Pein, Henry Von
Penick, Chester
Perez, Rolando
Perrin, Burt
Petry, John
Pharr, Odis
Philipp, Charlie
Phillips, Ed F.
Phillips, Ewart

Phillips, Joe
Pickle, J. J.
Picone, Joe Al
Pierson O. E.
Pigman, Jimmie
Pipes, Wayne
Poe, Thomas
Pope, Dan
Portele, J. R.
Poulan, H. K., Jr.
Powell, Elmon
Powers, G. T.
Powers, Melvin
Price, R. E.
Prince, Alvin
Prugel, A. E.
Puckett, Henry
Puig, Joseph
Raggio, C. J.
Ramirez, Marcelion
Ramsey, Clifton
Rankin, Harry
Raschke, William
Raska, Allan
Ray, W. E.
Redman, Joe B.
Reese, Martin
Reeves, Elbert
Reeves, George
Reid, Ernest L.
Reid, Wm. "Bill"
Renner, Ray
Rhoten, W. Don
Richardson, Gordon
Richardson, Wayne
Rickert, Bruce
Riley, D. Schley
Riley, Jack
Rister, E. P.
Rittimann, Edward
Roark, Chris
Robertson, Frank
Robinson, C. Don
Robinson, Frank
Robinson, J. W., Jr.
Robinson, Joe
Robinson, Sam
Rockett, Chad
Roe, H. Jack
Roeber, Walt
Rogers, Alfred
Rogers, Claude
Rose, Lindall
Ross, Jimmy
Ross, Sam
Roten, W. W.
Rubin, Morris
Runnels, L. E.
Rutherford, W. R.
Ryals, Felix
Ryan, E. L.
Rygaard, Pete
Sackett, Floyd
Sanchez, Nick
Santa Maria, Al
Santos, Alex
Sattler, Adam
Sayles, Robert
Schaefer, B. C.
Schlie, Robert
Schleider, Robert
Schmid, Al
Schneider, Clyde
Schneider, Leroy
Schroeder, Herbert
Schumann, H. L.
Schumann, H. T.
Schwab, John W.
Schwartz, Gene
Schwartz, M. M.
Schwartz, Milton B.
Schwethelm, A. C.
Scott, C. S.
Scott, Jesse
Scudder, Louis
Sebera, William
Secord, Charlie
Seelig, John E.
Self, R. A.
Shafer, R. A.
Shaffer, Ben
Shaffer, S. G., Jr.
Shaffer, Scurry, Jr.
Shamburger, Carl
Sharp, A. C., Jr.
Sharp, S. A., Jr.
Sharpe, Bob
Shely, Buster
Shepherd, H. H.
Sheppard, Stan

Sherman, Frank A.
Shock, Vernon
Shore, Orval
Shotwell, P. E.
Silverberg, Herb
Simpson, E. B., Jr.
Simpson, E. G.
Skelton, Howard
Slater, Bert
Slider, David
Sloan, Joe
Sloman, Wiley W.
Smith, Damon
Smith, F. T.
Smith, Floyd
Smith, Gordon
Smith, J. A.
Smith, James
Smith, Jere
Smith, Jesse
Smith, Larry
Smith, Noel
Smith, Otto, Jr.
Smith, Reagan
Smith, Roscoe
Smith, V. H.
Smith, W. L.
Smith, William A.
Smith, William J.
Snider, Marion B.
Snodgrass, N. K.
Snyder, Duane
Snyder, Howard
Sorrels, Tommy
Sparks, Bryan
Sparks, W. B.
Spence, George
Spencer, Ken
Spivey, Harold
Spradlin, Dwayne
Stamey, O. L.
Standard, Fred W.
Stark, Don
Starnes, H. L.
Steakley, Zollie
Steele, Jimmy
Stein, William
Stephan, E. A.
Stephens, J. M.
Stephens, Julius
Stephens, O. A.
Stevens, C. J.
Stevens, J. R.
Stevenson, Sid
Stevic, William, Jr.
Stewart, James
Stokes, A. D.
Stokes, Fred
Stout, Chester
Stover, J. L.
Stowe, Walter
Strange, Joseph
Strickland, George
Stripling, Cecil, Jr.
Strong, Jack
Stucke, Kenneth
Summers, Bill
Summers, Randy
Sutton, H. Gene
Sutton, Joe
Swanson, Lester E.

Tawwater, W. L.
Taylor, Don
Taylor, Robert
Teas, Don
Teggeman, Erwin
Templeton, Cecil
Thames, Ed
Thomas, Ralph R.
Thompson, B. R.
Thompson, G. E.
Thompson, George
Thornton, Fred
Tijerina, Ernesto
Tinkel, Jim
Tocker, Robert
Towerey, W. R.
Treadaway, Henry
Tremble, Al
Tribble, A. C.
Triplett, E. F.
Tuebe, Ewald
Tunnell, Pat
Tyler, Wm.

Van Camp, Virgil
Van Tyne, Gayle
Vandiver, Jerry
Vangel, Lous
Vaughn, Thomas
Von Roeder, Max

Vorhes, Joe J.
Waddle, P. H.
Walding, Jack
Wales, Bill
Walker, Albert
Walker, Gerald
Walker, Guy
Walker, H. Y.
Wall, David
Wallace, James
Wallace, James P.
Waller, Jim Ed
Ward, Chuck
Ward, James
Ward, John B.
Ward, Morris
Ward, Tom
Waters, Philo
Waugh, Kenneth W.
Waymire, Glenn
Weaver, Joe
Webb, Carlisle
Webb, Ralph
Webb, W. E.
Weis, George
Weiss, Erwin
Werner, Robert
Westbrook, Glendon
Wheeler, Billy
Wheeler, James C.
Wheeler, James H., Jr.
Whitaker, Pat S.
White, Harold
White, J. A.
White, Joe
White, Raymond
Whitlock, Lloyd
Wickersham, Harry, Jr.
Wicker, Dave
Wiech, Jack
Wiggins, C. F.
Wilburn, Theo
Wiley, Bill
Willems, George
Williams, Charles
Williams, Dr. Jay
Williams, J. S.
Williams, J. R.
Williams, R. J.
Willis, Darwin
Willis, Russell
Wilmoth, Paul
Wilroy, T. J.
Wilson, Charles
Wilson, Jim Bob
Wilson, W. Andrew
Windham, John
Winterfield, Ken
Wise, Jack
Wisehart, Harry, Jr.
Wishnow, Dr. Irv
Wofford, C. D.
Wolfe, C. M.
Wolters, Freddie
Wolverton, Steve
Wood, Bill
Wood, William
Woodson, Charles
Wooldridge, J. B.
Wooley, J. W.
Wooley, Roy
Wooster, Stoy
Word, David
Woytek, Lester
Wright, Harold
Wright, Jack
Wuensche, John
Yorfino, Joe
Young, Charles
Young, Raymond
Zimmerman, Don

— Chapter 11 —

"A Lion Never Rests"

"God bless these men. They must be good men because they love little children — even crippled ones."

— A Camper

Texas Lion Schutte put it this way: "If you owned a piece of property and paid the taxes, you'd go out there every once in a while to check on it, wouldn't you? It's the same way with our camp for crippled children. We, the Lions own it; we're proud of it. We all try to go out there once in a while and check on our investment." Executive Director Glenn Crawford said Lions and other visitors were always welcome and he had observed that once they saw the camp in operation "they were hooked for life."

Wearing yellow and purple baseball caps and the familiar vests increseted with the Lions Clubs International symbol, the statewide owners of the camp regularly arrived to check their investment and watch the children at play. Every spring they went to camp to do clean-up and repair work before summer camp opened. Sometimes they went with other Lions; sometimes they arrived alone or with their spouse. During the summer more Lions came because they loved to watch the children at work and play; the chil-

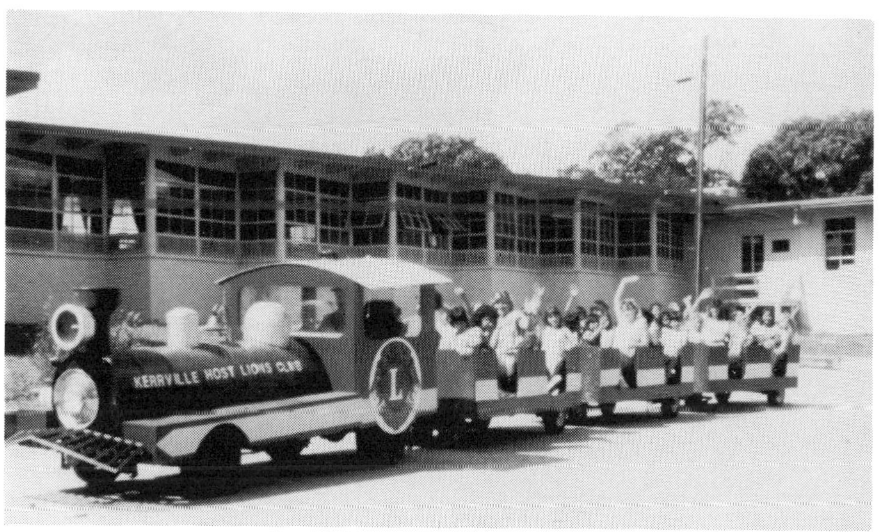

Kerrville Lions give campers a ride in their train.

dren loved it, too. Some of the Lions were tied emotionally to the children their clubs sponsored, and could not wait until the two weeks were up to check on their progress and happiness. In this case, most often that special child welcomed a much loved "Lion daddy or mother."

A parent of one handicapped boy said she "praised God" for these people who cared for special children and were willing to give of themselves. "My heart is touched. I had no idea the Lions did such a wonderful work. The camp will be in my prayers daily." A father said: "You didn't have to care. Seems not many people do. It's people like you who bring peace and joy to a hurting world. May God richly bless you and the camp. If there had been a fee my son couldn't have attended. I wish to try and send donations when I can. As God blesses me, I want to share it with you to meet the needs of special children like my son. It won't be much, but my prayers will make up the difference, I hope. I can never repay you for the love and care given. Please continue your work."

Thousands of Lions club members over Texas and their friends shouldered the entire camp operations. First, they gave specified portions of their annual dues toward camp expenses; then they planned, promoted, and sponsored some type of annual fund drive to raise more money. Next they assumed responsibility for contacting schools, doctors, and clinics to find children qualified to be campers; then they visited the parents to obtain permission to send their children. When sessions arrived, they packed up the children and transported them to camp; then they returned in two weeks on a Friday to attend the awards night, rooting for their special kids during awards-presentation. When it was over, they drove the happy children home. Crawford explained that many of these Lions traveled half way across Texas, and had to leave their businesses, but "they figure it's all worth it." One Lion member said when a person is not accustomed to seeing the handicapped children in action, they find it is amazing. He recalled the cute eleven-year-old boy with both legs missing. "He looked like a little frog in the water." Once a year every Lions club in the state saw a slide presentation of the camp, given by their elected director of the camp board. "That's when they dig in their pockets again," said Ron Anderson, director of development and public relations.

Texas Lions bragged about their camp, and backed it with action. They received international recognition for the promise they made to themselves decades ago. The camp's summer supervisor, Oscar Lopez, said he did not think the Lions realized the impact of their project on both the children and the counselors. He said it changed their lives. One parent was curious enough to figure out how much it cost the Lions to operate the camp. That particular year, he noted that it cost $47 per handicapped child and $83 per diabetic camper per day in that summer. He multiplied that by the number of children and days and came to the conclusion it cost the Lions approximately $1,133,900 to operate camp that summer. His note to the camp said "God bless you, all you people who give just because you care."

After four decades of successfully sponsoring the camp, the Lions thought up additional jobs for themselves. Districts decided to "adopt" the various buildings on the campsite, which meant that a district would be responsible for needed renovation of a certain building or would maintain air conditioning in a bunkhouse or be responsible for upkeep of the infirmary. Some of the districts dedicated their adopted building to individual members as a way of honoring that Lion.

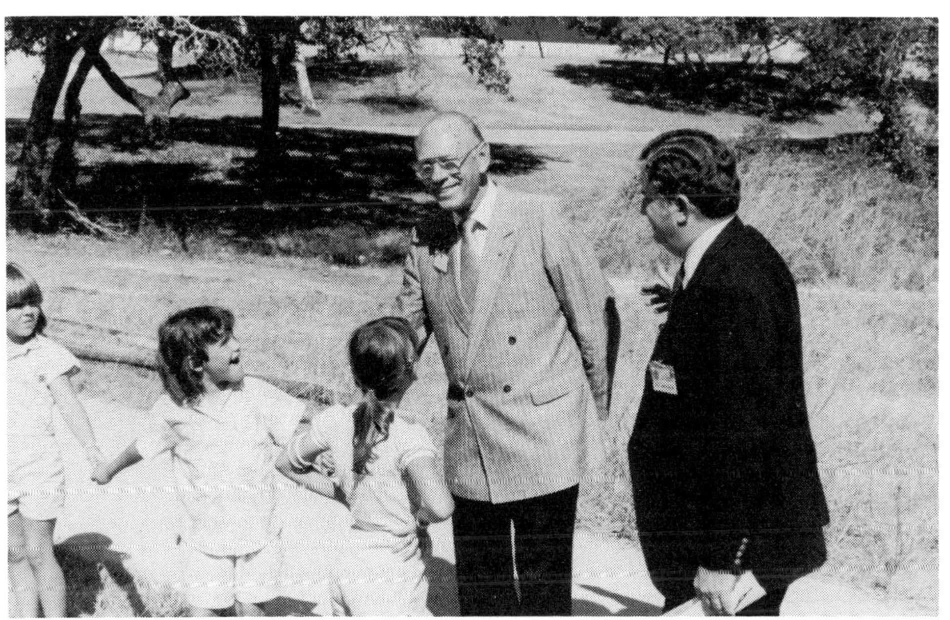

Sten Akestam of Stockholm, Sweden, left, past president of Lions International, visited Texas camp. At right was his guide, Ron Anderson, development director of the camp. It was a tradition for all international presidents to make an official visit to the Texas camp.

The individual clubs' fund-raisers each year were as wild as the games concocted by the kids at camp. There were turkey shoots, sheepdog trials, chili cookoffs, fish frys, pancake suppers, telethons, carnivals, womanless weddings, formal dances, horse shows. No one cared, as long as the money came in, but all ideas took time and work. One year the Alice Lions staged the "Great Tex-Mex Train Robbery" during which the Lions, dressed as *banditos* with big hats and guns, "held up" passengers. They captured them and charged them to be "shot" by a camera, with all proceeds going to the camp. Memorial Lions Club of Houston sold enough barbequed chickens to give the camp close to $2,000, while the Weslaco Lioness Club produced and sold a cookbook for almost an equal amount. Only rodeo bull riders of world standing were invited to a George Paul Superstar Bull Riding Contest in San Antonio in the mid-eighties which benefitted the camp. Paul was the only man in the world to ride seventy-nine consecutive bulls. This event was aired on national television and featured many entertainment stars.

Other projects have included a Cadillac auction by the Alvin Lions; a wild game supper in Livingston which had as dessert armadillo pie; tournaments such as golf, bowling, rodeo, and tennis; and games of all kinds, including football, basketball and soccer. When Abilene's annual charity football game between McMurray College and a guest team donated proceeds to the camp, Nolan Underwood, of the PR staff, accepted the money at half time. The cover of the charity game's program featured pictures of Lions camp children. The Lions Clubs in Abilene and in Bellaire each at separate times gave away a new home as a fund- raiser. The Bluebonnet Lions Club of Kerrville, chartered in April of 1988, had the distinction of being the only all-woman Lions Club in the state. Due to its proximity to the camp, they were to hold their annual fund-raiser as an entertainment for campers. They planned to hold a "no-show pet show" where pet owners were to send in pictures and a story of their pet entry. The Bluebonnet club sponsored this at one of the 1988 session's check-in days when activities were needed. Entertainment featured several obedience trainers and a blind man with his "three invisible Chihuahua dog guides." Lions paid for their birthdays at the New Braunfels Noon Lions Club. Members sent checks to the camp, contributing $1.00 for every year of their life.

One year New Braunfels Lions involved the entire community by stressing the enlistment of club members, businesses and individuals in the area as century club donors. Ron Anderson helped coordinate this plan, with assistance from Lions and others. On a statewide basis, Lions calendars have been sold, as well as Christmas cards, light bulbs, candy, coloring books, and the traditional mops and brooms to hustle money for camp operation. Benbrook Lions of Fort Worth held a statewide triathlon to raise money. Participants came from all over Texas, including Rick Bowman, a double amputee. Bowman, also was among those participating in the 1986 State Championship Biathlon. He was a Fort Worth lawyer who lost both legs on a Navy flight deck, and began entering triathlons to show that "people who are handicapped are not disabled; it just takes them longer."

In 1988 the Texas Basketball Festival in Kerrville looked as if it would become a tradition. Sponsored annually for several years

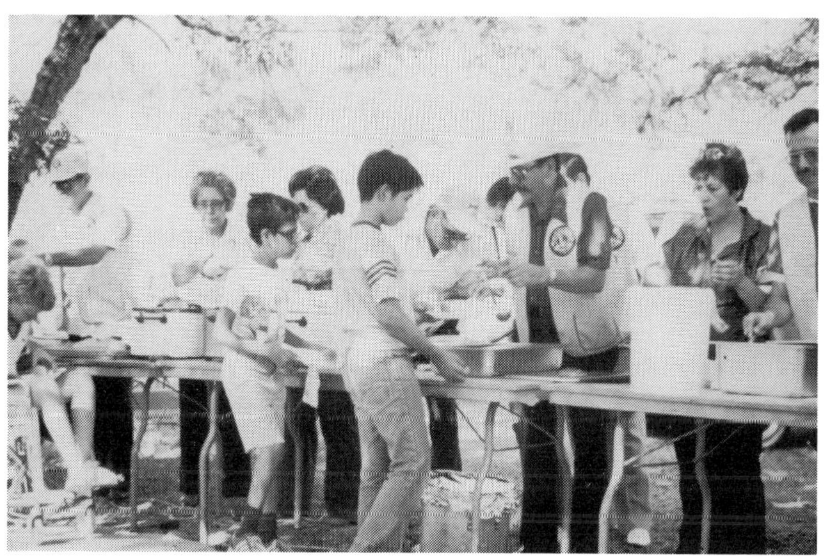

A Lions Club serves special meal at camp party.

by the Heart O' The Hills and the Host Lions Clubs in Kerrville, the event had gained momentum as top high school basketball teams gathered the last three days of the year. In 1987 over 5,000 people watched girls and boys teams play at Schreiner College and in Tivy High School gyms. Billed as the preview of the state basketball tournament, it was said that college scouts from several states attended the Lions games to recruit. All proceeds went to the children's camp.

Historically, the Brownsville Downtown Lions Club raised more money annually than most other clubs with its variety musical show which had been presented for over twenty-five years. Jack Wiech, one of the camp founders in 1949, was a member of this club. They worked all year long on the production, but it was no less important than the children of Lions in Childress one year who sold lemonade and sent all proceeds to the camp. One of the largest single donations of money from a Lions Club came from the Lubbock Club in the early eighties when they gave over $75,000 to build the second swimming pool.

The Laredo Evening Lions loaded up once every summer and

drove to camp to give a pinata party, a tradition which was almost as old as the camp. Industry West-End Lions paid for the Goodtimes Band to entertain the camp for a number of summers. One year the Graham Noon Lions Club brought a band for the awards night festivities at camp; Jacksboro Lions sponsored a band concert another summer, and they also gave a horse trailer to the camp.

In addition to dues and monies from fund-raisers, other items came in regularly, and usually unexpectedly, from individual Lions or from clubs, including such items as food, bedding, furniture, equipment, vehicles, and clothes. The Lake Brownwood Lioness Club raised their gift one year by collecting donations to the camp, then matching the amount they collected. The Killeen Lioness Club gave an enlarger and other darkroom equipment to camp, enabling the office to send photographs of the campers to their hometown newspapers; the Monahans Lions sent a calf to camp for fresh meat one year.

The declarations of Texas Lions Camp special "weeks" or "days" by governors for the State of Texas was always a "natural" for the Lions members to get busy and cash in on the promotion.

Lions helped in other ways. Those whose professions were in the economic realm were always available to give advice to the League, helping certain funds to make money. Lions in other businesses offered their special expertise when applicable. Crawford explained that all money donated "is carefully managed to provide the best services possible for the most children." A critical time in the Texas Lions camp history came in 1987 when the economic situation in Texas was reflected in camp donations. As a result, three hundred children in the handicapped camp and ninety children in the diabetic were turned away. No child had ever paid a penny to attend; and until that year, no child was ever turned away for lack of funds. Lions and their friends began working to see that such a situation never occurred again. The Rockdale Noon Lions Club assessed themselves an extra $10 per member to help alleviate this situation. Wrote Bill Cooke, editor of the *Reporter*: "If a person really wants to put things in perspective, he or she just needs to sit and watch an awards ceremonies at the end of one of those camp sessions. When it comes to achievement, Super Bowl and World Series heroes pale before the accomplishments of the camp youngsters."

The Lions organization was formed as a service club; its serv-

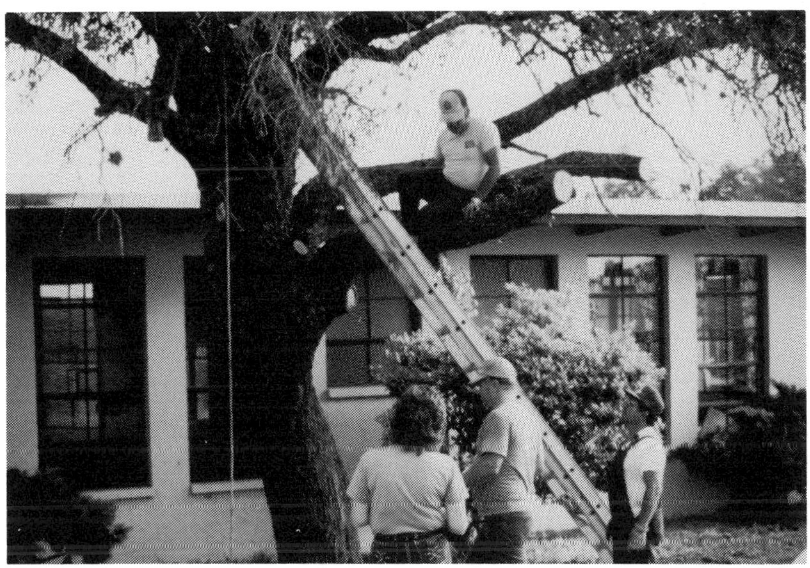

Lions and friends come from all over the state to clean up the camp and repair buildings and equipment before summer camp opened each year.

ices have encircled the globe. During World War II before the U.S. entered the conflict, the Lions' hearts in this nation went out to the orphans in England. In 1942, George Jordan of Dallas, read the following message from the Queen of Great Britain at the Lions Clubs International Convention in Toronto: "I am commanded to say that Her Majesty hopes you will convey her message to the Lions Clubs in their convention at Toronto for the generous gift of 14,000 pounds for the relief of the Waifs and Strays Society which Her Majesty appreciates very much."

In 1988, there were 40,279 Lions in Texas, belonging to 1,107 clubs. They took pride in the fact Lionism in Texas was recognized as the largest and most thoroughly organized service clubs in the U.S. The camp was their motivation unit. They felt deeply their vowed responsibility to be the champion for those tiny bits of humanity who could not help themselves. Lionism in Texas was not just another organization; it was a way of life, said Jack Wiech, a founder of the camp.

Randy W. Nickelson joined the Lions organization in 1988; a

safe hunter instructor, state-certified by the Texas Parks and Wildlife Department, he decided to spend his 1988 summer vacation as a volunteer at the camp. After his work there he told Lions and other friends that the name of the facility should be "Camp Love." He said "the comradeships and love between camper and staff is never ending." The first night of camp was reserved for welcoming ceremonies at which the stick ceremony was held. A classic Indian legend, the ceremony involved campers blowing their dreams into a stick, dropping it onto the fire, and letting their dreams scatter throughout camp in smoke. At the end of camp, they reported if their dreams or wishes had come true. Nickelson said he had a head cold at the time of the ceremony, but had made friends with a little boy. "When we got to the fire this young man, instead of wishing for his own well-being, asked that 'Mr. Randy's nose get better.' Fellow Lions, I do not know how high that smoke rose, but the next morning my head was as clear as it has ever been." He urged all Lion members who had not "seen this facility to plan an outing and experience real Camp Love."

The greatest tribute ever paid the camp or the Texas Lions, said Hyer in his fifty-year history of Texas Lionism, was given by one little girl who wrote and left this note in the pew at the camp chapel: "Thank you, dear Lord for the Lions of Texas who have made this camp possible for us crippled kids."

— Chapter 12 —

"It Takes Many Hearts"

"We know that by working with Texas Lions Camp, we are helping others. It allows us to pay a little rent on the space our Good Lord has allowed us to occupy on this earth."

— Ed Flood, past director Lions Clubs International

When parents, friends, the media, service groups, and others with compassionate hearts unite in a single cause, things happen. Walls crumble, spirits are healed, foundations built, and hope leaps forward. So it was with the Texas Lions Camp for Crippled Children.

The Lions knew they could have done it themselves, but from the very beginning of the idea in 1949, others wanted to help. Like the Lions, Lionesses and Leos, these citizens felt the camp would be one of Texas' greatest service facilities. They could see that it would fill a void in the lives of special boys and girls who just wanted to be as "normal" as possible. It was this compelling force that brought together many individuals, businesses and organizations. They were still helping in the camp's fortieth year, 1989.

Not since the first camper arrived one Sunday in 1953 had any child paid a dime for their stay at the camp. The Lions of Texas

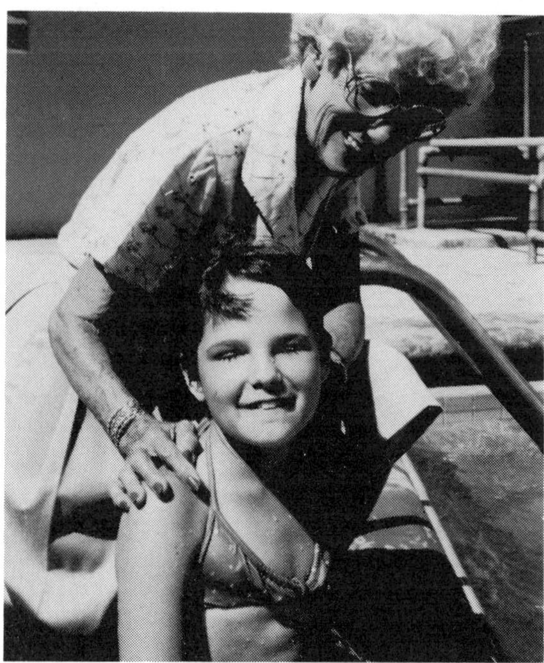

Harriet Kirby, Volunteer Coordinator, with camper at swimming pool.

supported the camp, but other people, especially parents, wanted to help. They were important help, too. A father of a camper wrote to the executive director: "I am most happy that my son has been given the opportunity to attend the camp to help improve his self-confidence and his interaction with other less fortunate children, and I would like to volunteer my time next spring when you begin the clean-up and preparations for the new season. I am well known to the working end of a paint brush, hammer, shovel or axe. And my back is strong as a bull! Please contact me when I may be of assistance."

Many parents spent every dollar they could collect on hospital bills and medical supplies for their handicapped children. This was why the Lions and their friends paid the camping bills. This was why so many mothers and fathers offered to help with repairs at the camp or sent small donations. They also helped to spread the word about the camp to other parents of children with disabilities. All were eager to tell of the benefits their son or daughter received at the Lions camp. This was important, because there had been times when the camp was not full and other children could have gone, if the Lions had just known where that child was.

Many individuals who heard about the camp and its rehabilitation program sent money, both in small amounts and in large donations. For many years, an anonymous envelope arrived once a month, without fail, and inside was a one dollar bill. On the other hand, the largest single donation from a non-Lion was when Victor Real willed the camp $275,000. This was used to construct Real Lodge for living accommodations. Ben Jackson, a Rotarian, gave $125,000 in the name of his sister, who had attended the blind program at the camp. This money, too, went to build Jackson dormitory/lodge.

One year the Fraternal Order of Eagles service organization selected the Texas Lions Camp as recipient of their statewide fund-raising project. A member of Eagle Aerie gave $5,000, pledging an additional $20,000. In all, that year the Eagles gave $65,000 to build the major nature trail for the children. The ground had to be leveled; the wide path curved and sloped. Railings were put at some spots along the path; at other places a wooden deck with attached benches was constructed. The bronze marker inlaid on a giant rock at the beginning of the long and beautiful trail identified the donors — the Texas State Aerie and Auxiliary, Fraternal Order of Eagles, in May 1985.

When the Lions of Texas agreed to build and operate the camp for handicapped children they knew it would be impossible without an abundance of promotion and publicity on a statewide basis. Here was where the media came in. Newspapers, magazines, television and radio stations all had cooperated with the Lions since the beginning. Untold amounts of newspaper and TV space had been devoted to publicizing the League's efforts to raise money and then to locate the campers.

It was almost a tradition — the media never said "no" to the Lions camp. In 1949 they splashed across their pages and airwaves the news that the League had been formed, and then again when it secured the camp site, and again when the camp first opened. Every year since, the media continued answering Lions' requests for help all over the state.

In 1987 the Texas economy almost hit rock bottom; and for the first time in the forty-year history of the Lions camp, children were rejected at the last minute because of lack of funds. The Hill Coun

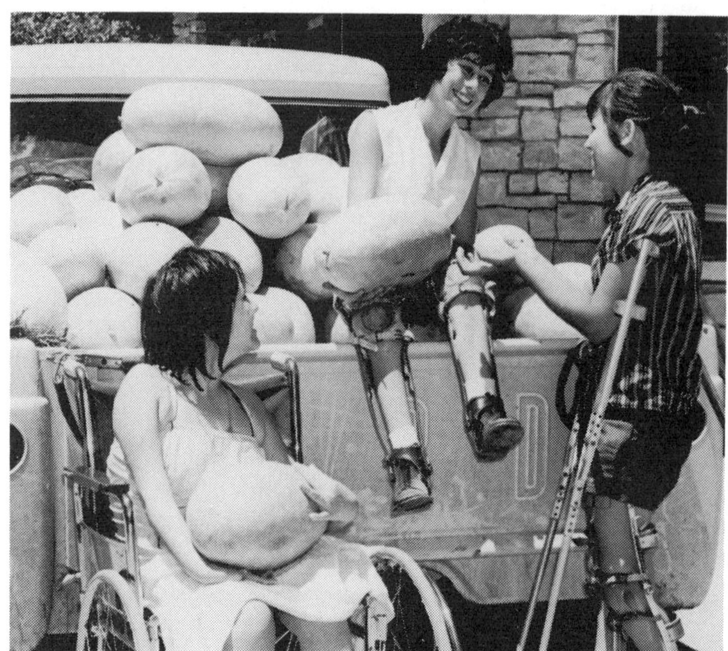

Campers love watermelon parties.

try Charity Ball Association in Kerrville vowed this would never happen again. Their annual benefit that spring was devoted to raising money for the children to go to camp. Included in the gala event were tennis tournaments, auctions, and the beautiful formal ball. The Association raised $42,000 for the camp. This campaign was entitled "Bring Back the Children," and did not end with the charity ball. Publicity about the event went throughout the state and precipitated numerous young people to produce service projects for camp funds. Among them were sixth-grade students at Notre Dame Catholic School in Kerrville who sent sixty dollars in cash, raised from a two-day bake sale.

Some of the items which individuals and groups sent to camp included deer meat from hunters, hunting clubs, and the state game department; truck loads of fruit and vegetables from the Rio Grande Valley; peaches and apples from nearby Stonewall. In one of the early years of the camp, the prize calf at the Houston Fat Stock Show, weighing 880 pounds, was donated by its purchaser. Many animals for slaughter were donated by 4-H Clubs in Kerrville and other parts of Texas. One year the Texas Parks and Wildlife Department stocked the one-acre lake on the campsite with 1,000 channel catfish and hybrid perch. They were fed from an automatic feeder donated by Lion A. J. Ruth. This made fishing popular at camp that summer.

For a number of years the annual National Milk Bowl benefited the camp. This was an invitational football game played by fifteen-year-old and younger boys who weighed one hundred pounds or less. It always received publicity, was highlighted by special appearances of persons in the entertainment field, and was covered by national sports broadcasters. Many Southwest Conference football officials volunteered their services.

McDonalds of Galveston one year sent their special cookies; the Two Sisters Antiques of Kerrville kept the camp supplied all one summer with videos for the children's entertainment. Another season the Hill Country Arts Foundation's Point Theatre Box Office in Ingram gave free show tickets to all children. Camp buses or vans took the campers to the nearby theatre. LaFours famous seafood restaurant in Kerrville for many years entertained some twenty campers and counselors at every session with their biggest seafood dinner.

A number of choral groups gave performances over the years. One such one was the Cypress Trail U.M.C. Children's Choir which came halfway across the state from Spring, Texas, paying their own expenses. In 1982 the U.S. Navy Seabees from Beeville built a beautiful log cabin for the camp which they named Campcraft. Special nature programs were held here. The Seabees also prepared a road and parking lot area for paving.

Small, but useful gifts, such as aquariums, TV sets, clothing, arrived at the camp headquarters often. W. C. DeWitt of Weslaco accompanied a child to camp one summer; and when he saw what was going on, he bundled up his years of work, a delightful seashell exhibit, and sent it to the camp. Due to his distinction as a seashell authority, this donation received nationwide attention.

The Heritage Creative Outdoor Advertising Company, headquartered in Austin, offered to place billboards in most Texas cities to publicize the annual Lions Camp Week, which was usually in November. Texas governors regularly declared this special week in a ceremony, and the media gave news of its observances.

Famous sculptor, C. W. (Chuck) Warden, donated a creation entitled "Laying the Trip" valued at $3,000 for a Lions League drawing. The bronze piece depicted a cowboy wrangler in his intense maneuver to "lay the trip" on an errant steer. One campers's grandfather gave himself. When he went to camp to pick up his grandson, he was so impressed, he went home and joined the local Lions Club and became one of its most active members that worked hard for the children's camp.

In the early days of the camp, a great deal of the material necessities were donated. By 1989 the nonprofit camp was in very stable condition financially, so when a truck or new picnic tables or dishwasher for the kitchen were needed, the League's purchaser took written bids for it. If a large amount of money was needed for a new building, perhaps, the League called on Ron Anderson, director of development. He was knowledgeable in fund-raising and applying for special grants from foundations and corporations. This involved talent in grant-writing, public relations, and developing new ideas for fund-raising.

J. I. Moore of Kerrville, who was one of the two living founders of the League in 1989, said he believed if people would just go out and see the camp in action, many, many private donations would come pouring in. Tall and stately, Moore was as alert as ever in trying to get those dollars into the camp. It was that way with him forty years ago; it would always be that way with him.

Mrs. Effie Robinson, who with her husband, W. L., handled the accounting for the camp, agreed with Moore. A Lioness, she hoped that some day the camp would hold annual open houses, so that people could see for themselves the good work done there. At her suggestion, Mrs. Robinson's Lioness Club had a policy of buying a life membership at $100 when a new member had been in the club for one year and one day.

Moore remembered when the League collected that first $100,000 to gain title to the camp site, and "there was not a dollar left for a bunkhouse. We just had to go out and start all over again." Retired from the Charles Schreiner Company, Moore kept a wary eye at all times for people who could easily write the camp into their wills.

Special camp dreams had been realized, year after year, because of people over the state who cared and who were generous. Crawford said that when one dream was fulfilled, another one seemed to pop up just ahead, take form and summon the Lions attention. "But, then there is no end to compassion and generosity,

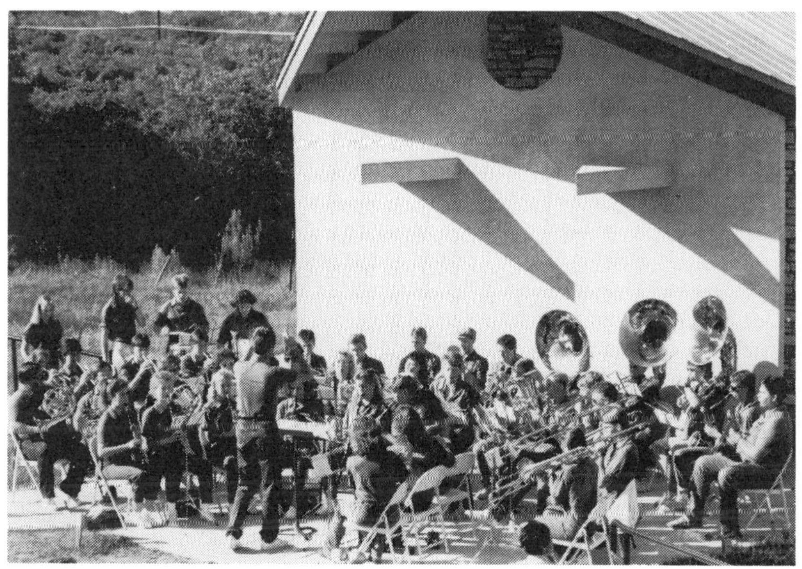

State Lions Band, composed of youngsters from every district in Texas, entertain campers at Amphitheatre.

just as there is no end to Texas Lionism," said Mrs. Robinson. "It always took the combined efforts of the Texas Lions and their friends, and the campers and their parents."

This column written by Erma Bombeck for the Field Newspaper Syndicate, was printed in newspapers on May 11, 1980.

> Most women become mothers by accident, some by choice, a few by social pressures and a couple by habit.
>
> This year, nearly 100,000 women will become mothers of handicapped children. Did you ever wonder how mothers of handicapped children are chosen?
>
> Somehow I visualize God hovering over earth selecting His instruments for propagation with great care and deliberation. As He observes, He instructs His angels to make notes in a giant ledger.
>
> "Armstrong, Beth, son, patron saint, Matthew. Forrest, Marjorie, daughter, patron saint . . . give her Gerard. He's used to profanity."
>
> Finally, He passes a name to an angel and smiles, "Give her a handicapped child."

The angel is curious. "Why this one, God? She's so happy."

"Exactly," smiles God. "Could I give a handicapped child to a mother who does not know laughter? That would be cruel."

"But has she patience?" asks the angel.

"I don't want her to have too much patience or she will drown in a sea of self-pity and despair. Once the shock and resentment wears off, she'll handle it.

"I watched her today. She has that feeling of self and independence that is so rare and so necessary in a mother. You see, the child I'm going to give her has his own world. She has to make it live in her world and that's not going to be easy."

"But, Lord, I don't think she even believes in you."

God smiles. "No matter. I can fix that. This one is perfect. She has just enough selfishness."

The angel gasps, "Selfishness? Is that a virtue?"

God nods. "If she can't separate herself from the child occasionally, she'll never survive. Yes, here is a woman whom I will bless with a child less than perfect. She doesn't realize it yet, but she is to be envied. She will never take for granted a 'spoken word.' She will never consider a 'step' ordinary. When her child says 'Mama' for the first time she will be present at a miracle and know it! When she describes a tree or a sunset to her blind child, she will see it as few people ever see my creations.

I will permit her to see clearly the things I see: ignorance, cruelty, prejudice, and allow her to rise above them. She will never be alone. I will be at her side every minute of every day of her life because she is doing my work as surely as she is here by my side."

"And what about her patron saint?" asks the angel, his pen poised in midair.

God smiles. "A mirror will suffice."

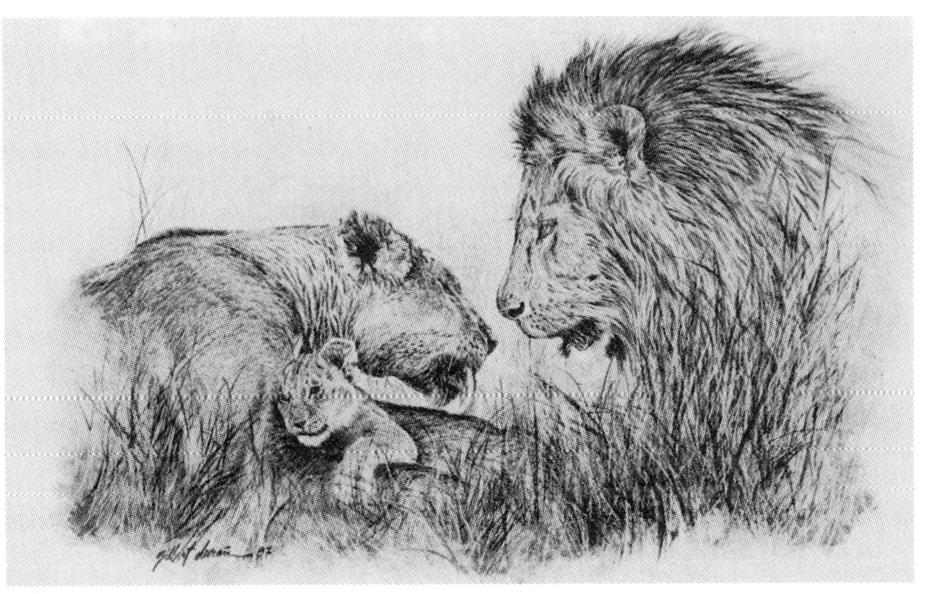

Lion's Pride by Gilbert Duran

— Chapter 13 —

"Grassroots of the Camp: The Staff"

"Your Texas Lions Camp prepares handicapped children to face the challenge of life and have a wonderful outdoor experience!"

— Ron Anderson, camp development and public relations director

Hurricane Gilbert hit the Texas Gulf Coast in mid-September, 1988, and recklessly moved inland. The staff at the Texas Lions Camp cancelled their usual working days to volunteer on an around-the-clock basis to assist in helping refugees fleeing from the storm. The camp was an American Red Cross-designated evacuation center, and a Red Cross emergency team went to the camp for an organizational meeting. Soon the staff welcomed over 325 evacuees from the Texas coastal area. The camp cook kept good food in the kitchen twenty-four hours a day, and program staffers held entertainment for the children refugees who came with their families. Staffers fielded this job with as much enthusiasm and ease as they did for the hundreds of handicapped children who romped over the grounds each summer and for the many senior citizens, school children and groups that convened there in winter for learning and fun.

The timeworn words, "It's all in a day's work," were some-

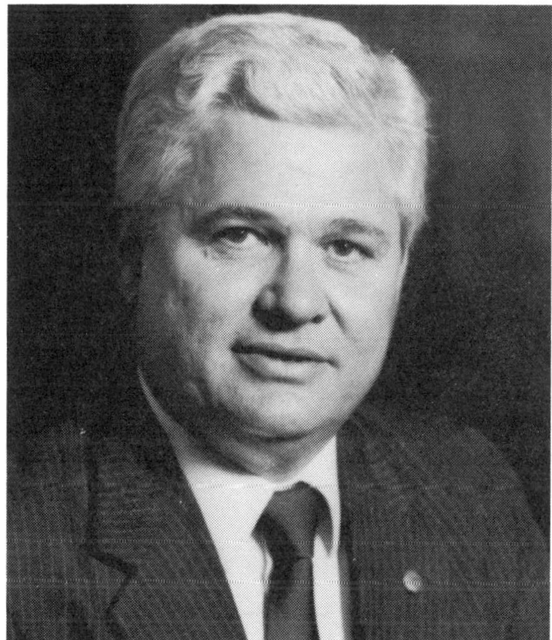

Glenn Crawford, executive director of Lions camp.

what more meaningful for the Texas Lions Camp staff than the average working person. There were not too many men and women whose daily jobs had the singular purpose of keeping alive a facility founded to rehabilitate, educate, and entertain handicapped children.

A normal day for Executive Director Glenn Crawford might have begun at 8:15 A.M. During one such day he held nineteen personal conferences or interviews; talked on the telephone to twenty callers; returned eight telephone calls; dictated eighteen letters; held a staff meeting; and read the daily mail which included district newsletters, newspaper clippings regarding Lions activities, general correspondence, and junk mail. He took about thirty minutes for lunch, and decided to leave the office at 7:15 P.M. to get a hair cut. Crawford's telephone calls involved such things as the computer system at the camp, purchase of a van, a club asking about roofing a bunkhouse, plans for a new administration building, IRS questions regarding donations to camp, a wide variety of fund drive plans over the state, and the list went on. Interviews concerned such things as care of a new horse, the Elderhostels, electrical problems in a camp building, approval of certain League bills, a ten-year reunion for counselors, and the list went on.

Sometimes his days were busier. Crawford might have driven to a Lions club meeting at noon or in the evening, either visiting or giving a speech/presentation. He might have decided to crank up the front-end loader and clear a ditch in front of a bunkhouse, drive a van full of sightseers over the camp, take directors to a firelight ceremony at Inspiration Point, or pack for a trip to Tennessee to bring back a horse that was donated to the camp.

During the summer camping season most days were busier because there were more visitors. Lions who brought children from over the state, or just went for a visit, all want to see him. Regardless, Crawford handled the Lion-owners of the camp, who were his employers, as expertly as he did the IRS. His stance was one of quiet, but forceful leadership, topped by good humor and plenty of ability.

The executive director holds a B.S. in biology-education and an M.Ed. in administration from the University of North Texas. He had almost enough hours from work at other universities to obtain doctorates in several fields: education, rehabilitation counseling, and administration, with a concentration of study in nonprofit administration. He had given seminars and workshops on rehabilitation and recreational programs for the blind and physically handicapped over the nation to many varied groups. Listed in Who's Who in both health care and state government, Crawford had worked with the Texas and Colorado state legislatures and rehabilitation administrations, as well as the Federal Rehabilitation Administration in various programs for the handicapped. He joined the Texas Lions League as executive director in 1978.

Records show that during his tenure, the number of handicapped children served in summer programs increased by thirty-four percent; the physical plant was expanded and improved over fifty percent of acquired cost of facilities; expenditures were maintained at twenty-eight percent below the consumer price index; and the program was expanded to international recognition. Crawford initiated staff training programs, developed the Outdoor Education Center into a year-around program, and reorganized the administrative and program staff for better client service delivery while reducing both staff cost and staff requirements.

Crawford inspired enthusiasm on the part of the staff regard-

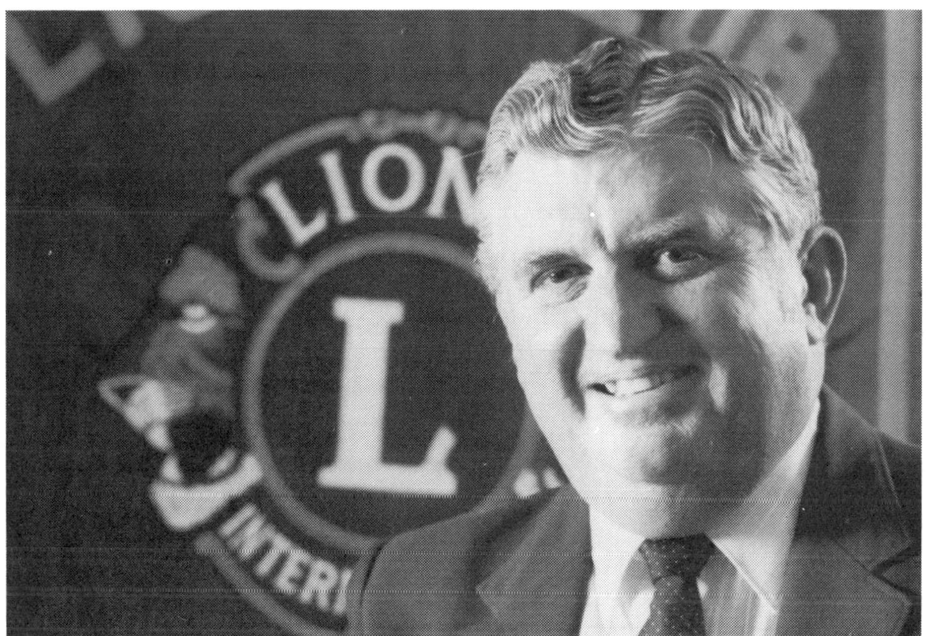

Ron Anderson, director of development and public relations.

ing the general service concept of Lionism, so that all members of the staff actively participated as members of Lions and Lioness Clubs. He required of his staff that they be very knowledgeable in their areas of responsibility.

"A high level of professional skill must be demonstrated by every camp employee," he said. "I have worked as a professional in rehabilitation for twenty-two years, eighteen of which was in administration. The ability of the camp's staff equals any with which I have been associated. In addition, rehabilitation staffers must be caring persons with concern for the well being of others. My staff measured up in all respects, and exceeded the anticipated in most."

Executives just below Crawford in authority and responsibilities were Ronald "Ron" Ray Anderson, director of development and public relations; Rand Southard, program director; Eleanor Toops, office manager; and Don Barnes, operations director.

Anderson held a B.A. and masters degree in biological sciences from Baylor University, and had worked toward a doctorate at the University of Arkansas. In addition he received certification in financial development and planned giving from courses he took at Colorado State University, Southern Methodist University in Dallas, and San Antonio. He attended the Singer Corporation's master marketing training program in New York City. Anderson had given seminars on development and outdoor training programs throughout the nation, and was a nationally recognized expert on early Texas history, treasure hunting, and fishing. He was a certified NRA instructor for rifles, handguns, and shotguns. Past employers included Follett Educational Corporation, Texas Parks and Wildlife Department, W. R. Grace Educational Products, and Temple, Texas, Independent School District. His work at the Lions Camp took him over the state frequently to make speeches and slide presentations; and in addition, he was the camp's professional fund-raiser and public relations consultant.

Southard, a certified camp director of the American Camping Association, held a BS in elementary education and special education from the University of Texas, Austin, and an ME in educational administration from Southwest Texas State University. He was appointed camp program director in 1983. The first full time program director was John Roper of El Paso who served the camp from 1961 until 1964, and again from 1968 to 1981. Other persons had served as program director but never in a full time capacity.

Barnes joined the Lions Camp in April of 1985, and as operations director he directed the dining hall, all maintenance and improvements of building and grounds, and janitorial services. He spent eight years in the navy and was assistant foreman of the plumbing department at Stephen F. Austin University in Nacogdoches, Texas, for seven years. At one time he spent eight years as camp director/ranger for a Boy Scout camp in north Texas.

Toops, a native of Florida, moved with her family to Kerrville after her husband, Paul, retired from a navy career. She began work as office manager for the Lions Camp in 1981, and said she was "grateful for the opportunity to be a small part of the great work carried on by the Lions and Lionesses of Texas. Working here at the camp is one of the most enjoyable and rewarding experiences of my life." She described Crawford as a "patient, kind and caring person who gives untold hours of constant vigil and dedication to the camp."

Staff members in the administration office, in addition to Crawford, Anderson and Toops, were Nolan Underwood, Tim

Hayes, M. A. Crawford, Linda Barnes, Toni Ashwood, Debbe Kegin, Wilma Hudson, and Nelda Dean. Ashwood was daughter of the late Jack Roe, whose idea was the basis for creating the camp.

The program office was under the direction of Southard, who said of Crawford: "He brought two important things to the camp when he came as executive director — growth and professionalism. It is phenomenal how the camp has grown and how it has been turned into a professional operation since Glenn arrived. Serving under Southard were Mae Nell Rhymes, who with twenty-six years on the staff had the longest tenure of any camp employee; and Oscar Lopez, Chris O'Quinn, Keith Smith, Mike Lackey, Jennifer Grace (a university intern), and Greg Holcomb.

Joe Haren was camp printer; and maintenance staffers included Dean Atkins, Brian Atkins, Bobby Gore, Carolina Pruneda, and Fabian Garcia. Assisting Thomas Andrysiak, food service manager, were Jodi Newell and Mark Hunt, permanent employees. During the summer the camp had as many as fifteen kitchen helpers. "Permanent" volunteers included Peggy Underwood, Erich Arnold, and Betty Arnold.

Camp employees and their families who lived on the campgrounds were the Crawfords, Andersons, Southards, and Barnes. Living in staff lodges were Lopez, Garcia, Grace, and Holcomb.

The first executive director and second president of the League was Frank Robertson, who had been a member of the Alamo Heights Lions Club in San Antonio where he was a builder/developer. Before accepting the position and giving up his work in San Antonio, he was afraid "it might be too depressing, but at the camp the depressed feeling turned to enthusiasm almost immediately." He served the camp for twenty-three years. Robertson said of the campers, "We just let them be as normal as they could. They went on overnight hikes and camped out like any other youngsters." The children loved him, and many identified with him because he was losing his eyesight when he became the director. He could be seen about the campgrounds making his way expertly with the traditional white cane.

Next director, who served for three years, was J. L. McPherson, a League president from 1975–77. McPherson was a retired personnel executive with Southwestern Bell when he accepted the appointment. He informed the directors he could serve only two or three years, while they searched for a permanent director. His

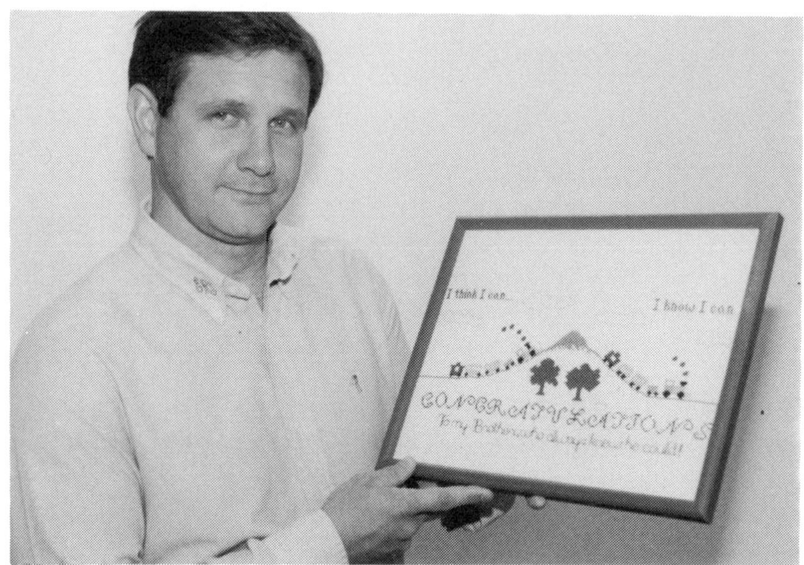

Rand Southard, camp program director, with a needle-worked picture his sister created. It said "I think I can, I know I can." Rand, an amputee, was a camper and counselor before joining the permanent camp staff.

leadership was so successful that he had to remind the directors at the end of his second year to start looking for someone else. His major achievements included development of written personnel policies, organization of staff into a systematic structure by programs, and providing badly needed repairs and maintenance of existing facilities.

Kids in summer camp always tried to hitch a ride on the mechanized carts used by most maintenance men and a number of staffers. "When we would let them ride," laughed Barnes, "then they would try to outdistance our carts in their wheelchairs." He once said that the way those kids whizzed around camp, the wheelchairs became "lethal weapons." Numerous times during any summer the maintenance staff was asked to repair broken crutches and wheelchairs; most orthopedic equipment had to be sent to specialists, said Barnes.

One summer counselors asked campers to fill out a little questionnaire. One question asked was "What I like best about the

Lions Camp?" A little girl named Mary Jane answered: "Nolan Underwood for solving my problems." Underwood was in the public relations department of the administrative staff, and had a masters degree in psychology and was a state certified counselor. Sometimes the program staff or counselors called on him to solve a behavior or emotional problem with a camper.

Underwood did a great deal of speaking and giving slide presentations over the state at Lions club meetings. After an appearance with Ron Anderson at a meeting of Lions in White Oak, Texas, J. Harold Spivey, the district governor and state Leo chairman, wrote this letter: "What can I say, guys? You were super! The kids were spellbound with your presentation. I just love to listen to lectures about our camp. Every time I do, I learn something new. The Lions of Texas are very fortunate to have such fine individuals as yourselves working there at the Texas Lions Camp. Your hard work and dedicated devotion shows. May I, as one of the 40,000 Texas Lions, say 'thank you and may God bless you for your efforts'."

Crawford required all staffers to be flexible, as they might be called upon to give a tour of the camp or visit with parents. They were required to have accurate information on Lionism in general and the Texas camp in particular. Crawford said he wanted all visitors at the camp to leave with very positive feelings.

Food Service Administrator Andrysiak, who had a degree in culinary arts, tried to make the kitchen a part of the camp. When the kids held parades, his kitchen crew dressed in costume and joined the festivities. He devised a system of giving each wing of a bunkhouse two tickets daily. The wing leaders were asked to give the tickets to kids who had been special helpers. The ticket entitled the bearer to extra dessert that night or ice cream. Andrysiak said he was training his kitchen staff to become real chefs. The kids always asked him, "Thomas, what surprise do you have for us today?" A mute child in one summer session took a special liking to Thomas. Each morning the boy came to breakfast and first made a "mustache" sign, which was his way of asking for Thomas. Seeing him, he gave Thomas a big "good morning" hug.

A number of husband-wife staffers served in the camp over the years. Buddy Murray of Kerrville was a maintenance supervisor for nearly two decades, and at times his wife, Vera, was responsible for the kitchen. For numerous summers, the night switchboard op-

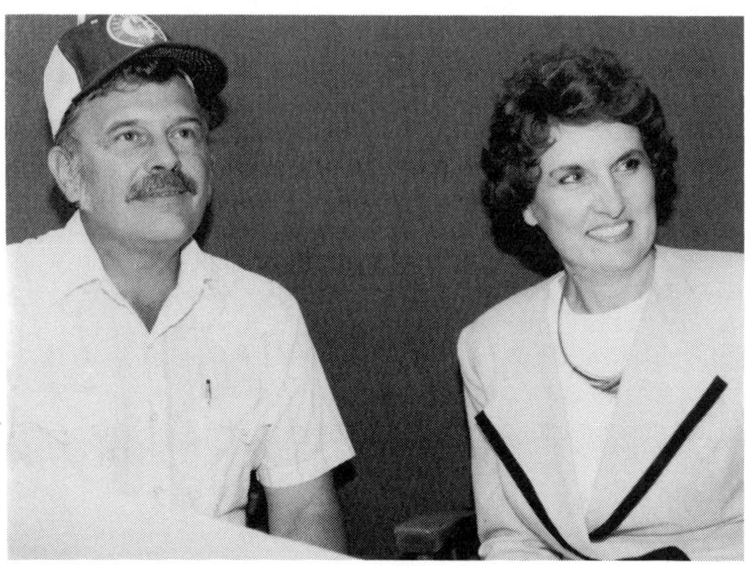

Don Barnes, left, was operations director, and Eleanor Toops was office manager at camp.

erator was Dann Kirby, who was blind and came all the way from El Paso because he loved the camp. His wife, Harriette, headed the volunteers who helped out in numerous ways during the summers. Sometimes there were as many as 150 volunteers. She also taught dancing to the campers. Dann used Braille, cassette tapes and an electronic computer to answer the telephones. Another blind employee of the camp was George McGonagill, who worked at the camp from 1957 to 1987 as a teacher in the winter blind program and in several other capacities. He retired to live in Kerrville, but returned when needed to help Joe Haren in the camp printing shop. His wife Judy was a teacher in the Camps training for adult blind persons.

Crawford's wife, M. A., did all the typesetting for camp printing projects, as well as designing layouts for newsletters, posters and the other promotional materials. Haren joined the camp staff in 1982 and began the print shop using one small "hand-me-down" machine, he explained. His work was outgrowing camp facilities in 1989, like all the camp areas, and he was planning to move the printing shop into the old administration building when the new one was constructed. He was just waiting for room and installation of modern equipment already donated. Haren said the camp material was important because many of the 50,000 Lions and friends who received it had never visited the camp, and were continuously amazed at the vastness of the facility. The print shop could not handle full color printing work in 1989, so that part of the Lions material had to be sent out. Haren waited for the day when he, too, would be able to produce Lions work in living color.

All money donated to the Texas Lions camp for handicapped children was carefully managed by Crawford and his staff in order to provide the best possible services. Crawford and Texas Lions believed that their camp was tops among all such facilities. As when the camp first began, Crawford added that "we are exceeding all expectations in every area."

One parent wrote saying, "My son has really changed his attitude since he started going to your camp. He has also become more responsible. I don't know how else to say thank you. It is people like you that give our children a good life." Another mother stated that the camp was "a wonderful place with great people working there and running it."

The camp received this note: "As a first-time camper's parent, I would have liked to have seen more of the camp grounds, facilities, cafeteria, and met the counselors. I would have enjoyed awards night, but I couldn't afford motel accommodations for overnight. Slade enjoyed the food. Thanks to all of you for a wonderful first-time camping experience for my son." The following year Lions in Slade's hometown saw that both he and his mother got to camp, with accommodations and plenty of time to see the facility that so changed her son.

Almost every evening, when the sun dropped behind the western hills like a big orange balloon and Crawford locked the office door, he looked up toward Inspiration Point with a satisfied feeling. His staff had gone home that day with a "job well done" for the crippled children of Texas; and as far as he was concerned, that was being almost to heaven.

Presidents of the League

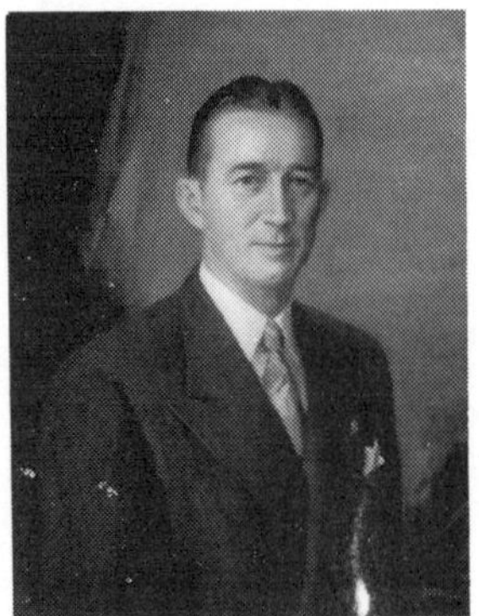

Jack Wiech
1949–52

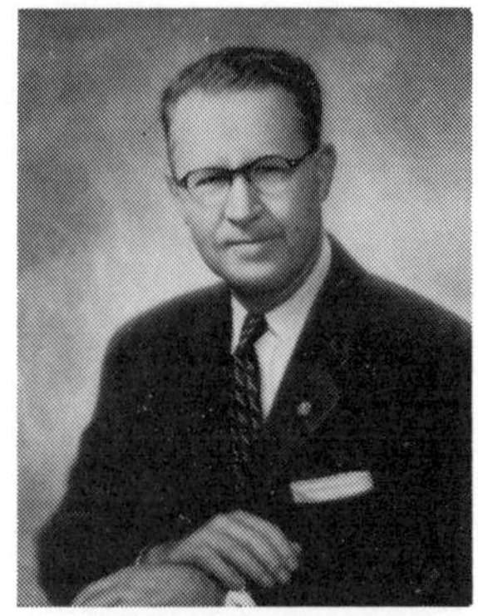

Frank Robertson
1952–56

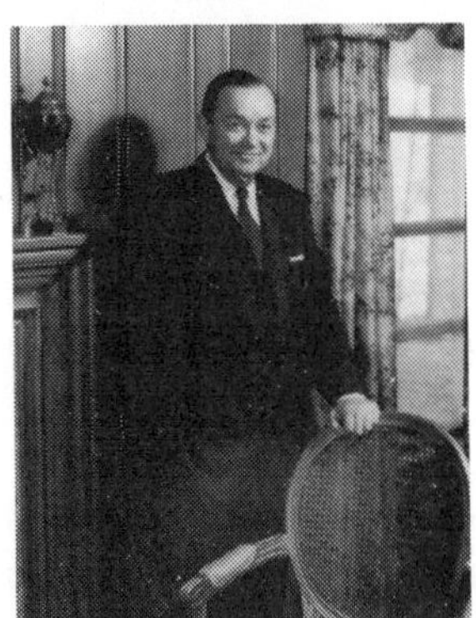

Reagan Smith
1956–60

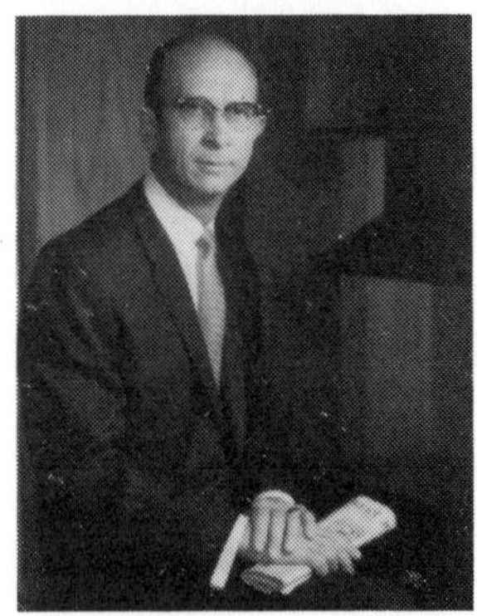

Jim Ed Waller
1960–65

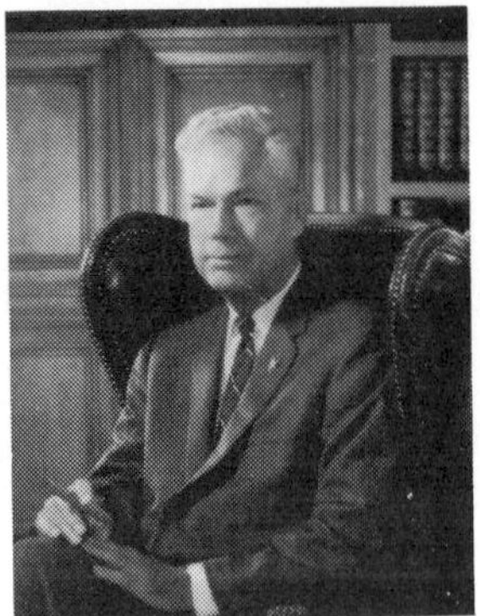

Roland C. Jordan
1965–67

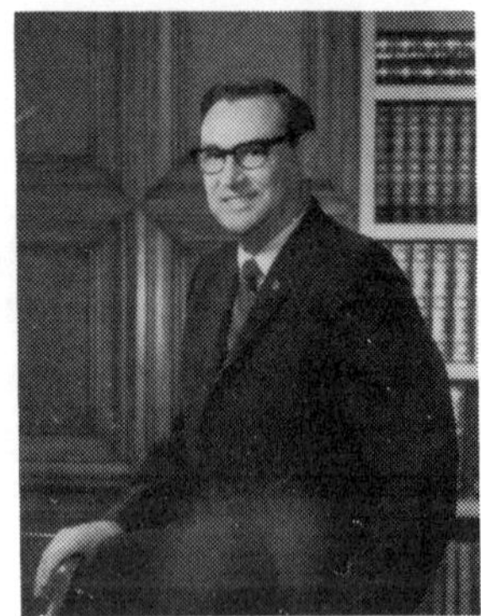

E. H. Munger
1967–69

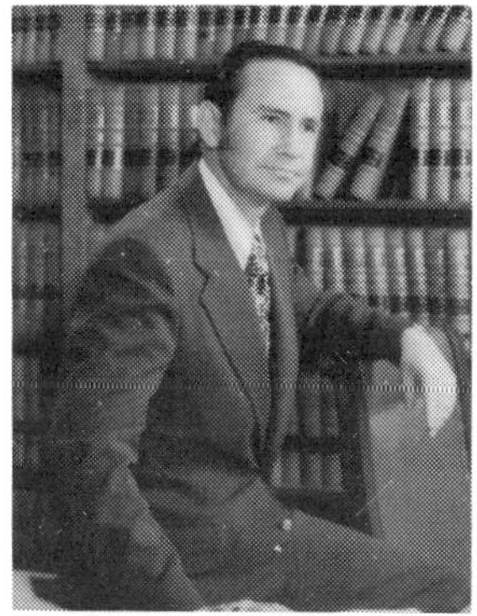

E. J. Grindstaff
1969–71

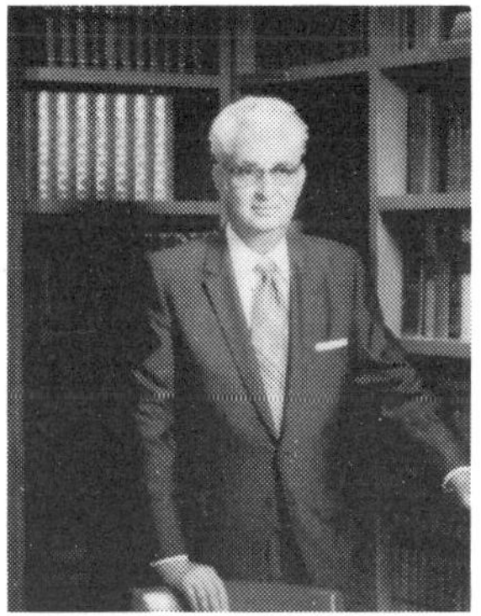

J. P. McCracken
1971–73

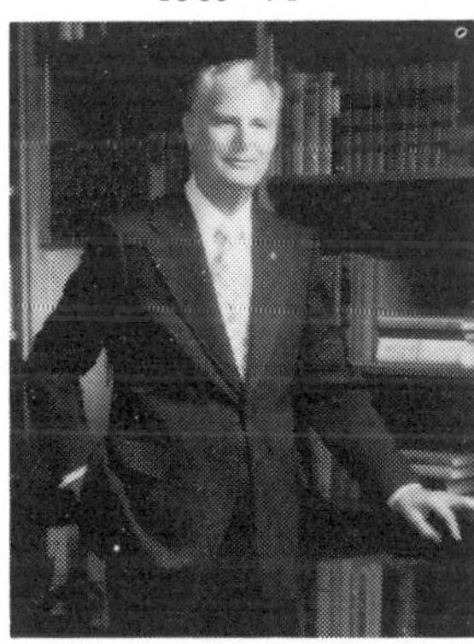

J. L. McPherson
1973–75

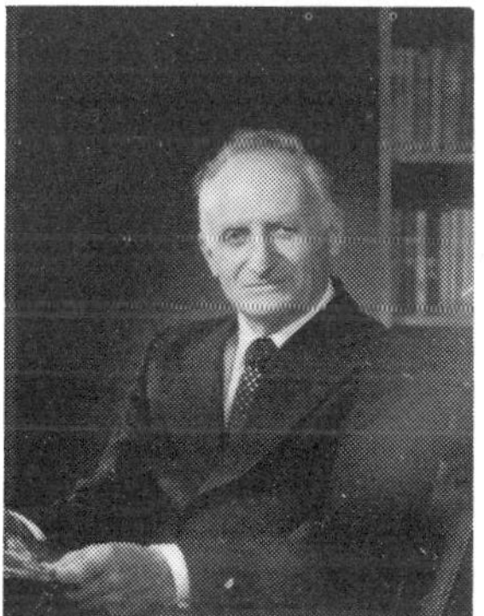

Sam Pakan
1975–76

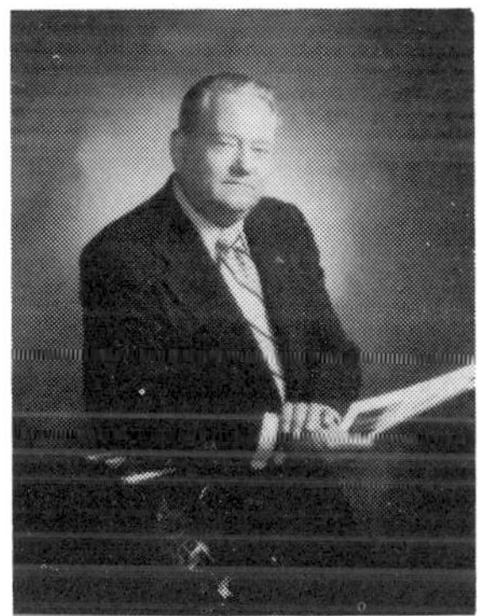

James Ward
1976–77

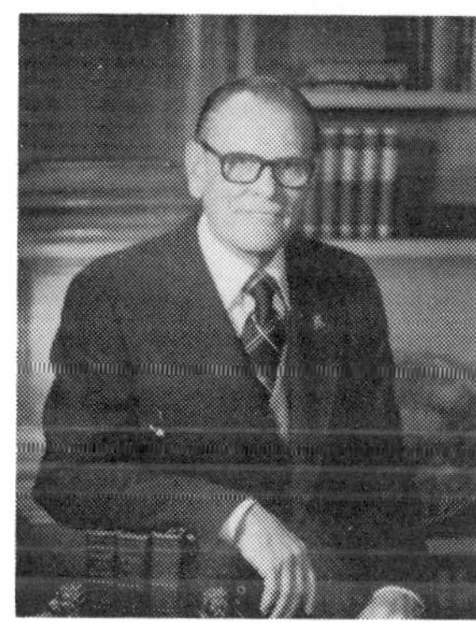

Herbert F. Barsh
1977–79

Presidents of the League

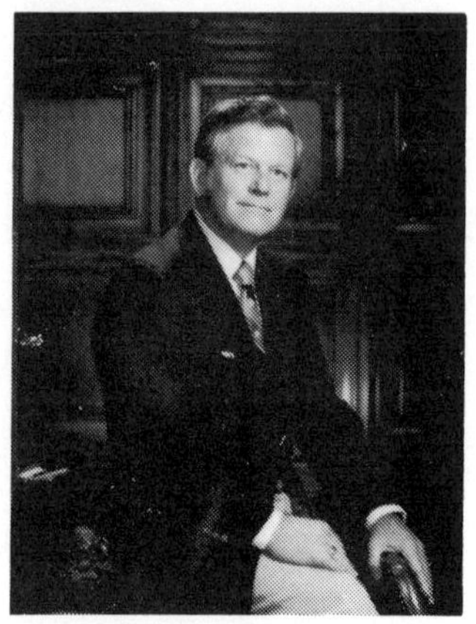

James H. Wheeler, Jr.
1979–81

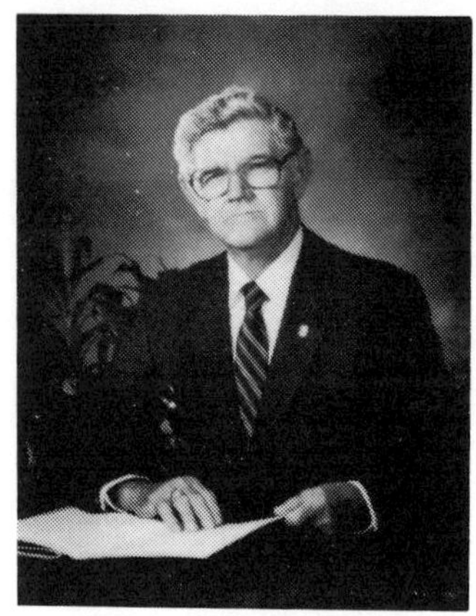

Fred Hamilton
1981–83

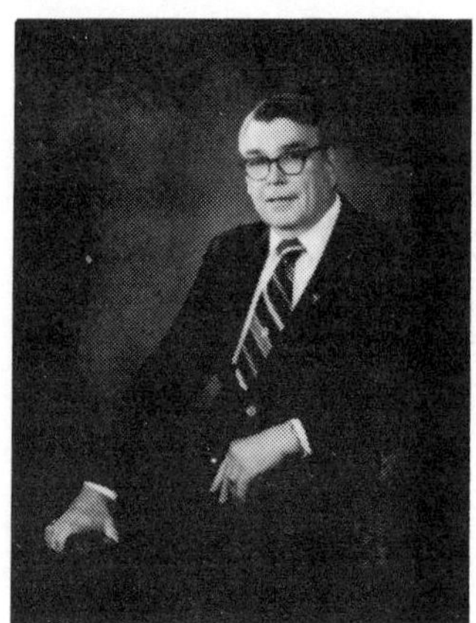

R. E. Price
1983–84

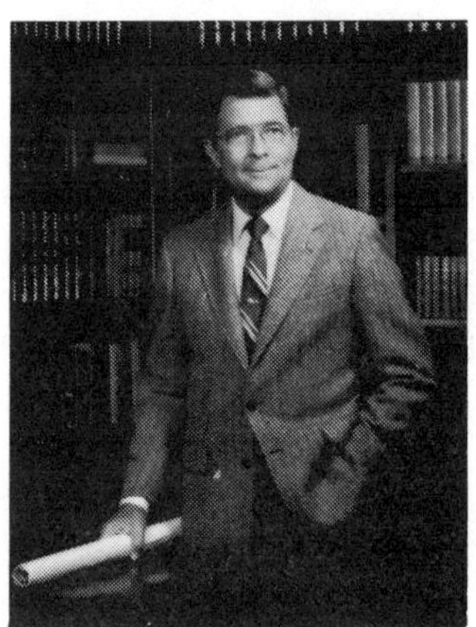

Roy N. Davis
1984–85

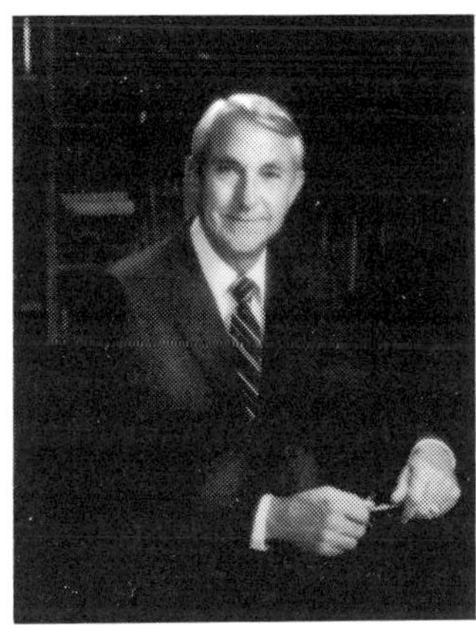

Raymond White
1985–86

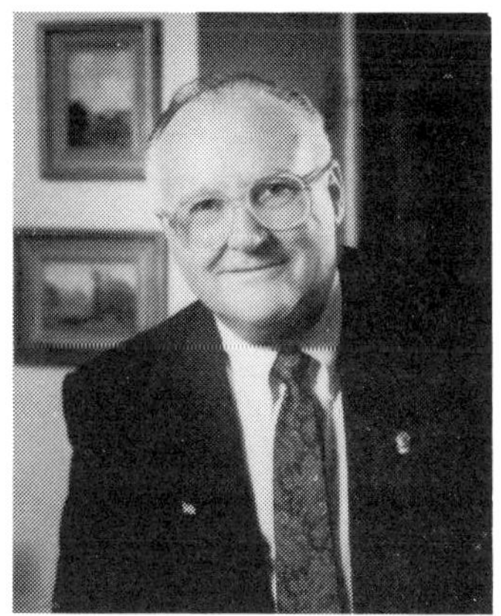

J. L. Akridge
1986–87

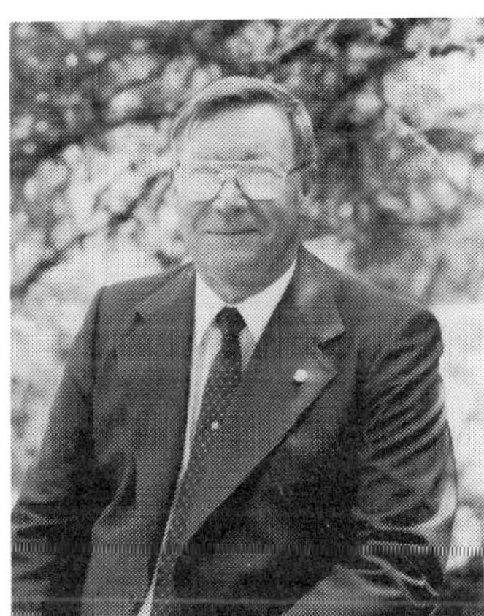

Marshall Cooper
1987–88

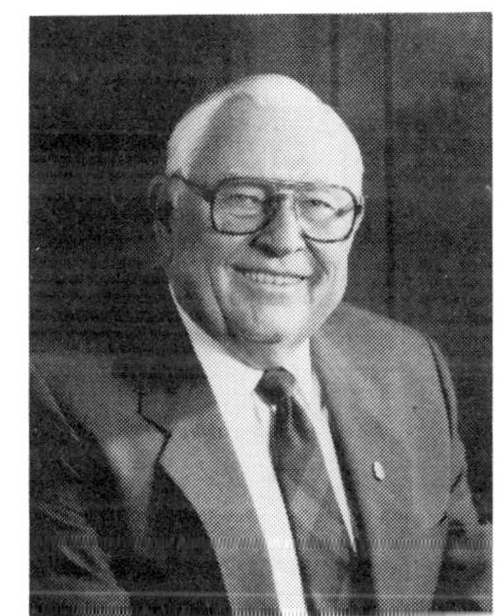

F. Ray McLaughlin
1988–89

— Chapter 14 —

"White Cane Club"

"Lou Etta could find her way in the dark, day or night"
— A Counselor

Arthur hailed a taxi in Houston, got in and gave his address. The driver could not find it, so Arthur directed as best he could. That turned out futile, too. Finally the impatient driver turned around to look at Arthur and was surprised to see he was blind. "If I'd known you were blind, I wouldn't have picked you up," he said rudely. Arthur answered: "And if I'd known you were so dumb I wouldn't have gotten in this cab!"

Arthur had been a football player and star black athlete who was blinded by an accident in his thirties. He became bitter and resentful toward life. A counselor referred him to the Texas Commission for the Blind. Reluctantly, after many unhappy days, he went to the commission's office in Houston. They sponsored Arthur for personal adjustment training at the Texas Center for the Blind at the Lions camp near Kerrville.

High on a hilltop, where the birds sang and the wind whispered through the trees and into the canyons, Arthur found something his soul needed, peace. He found another thing, too, hope. He

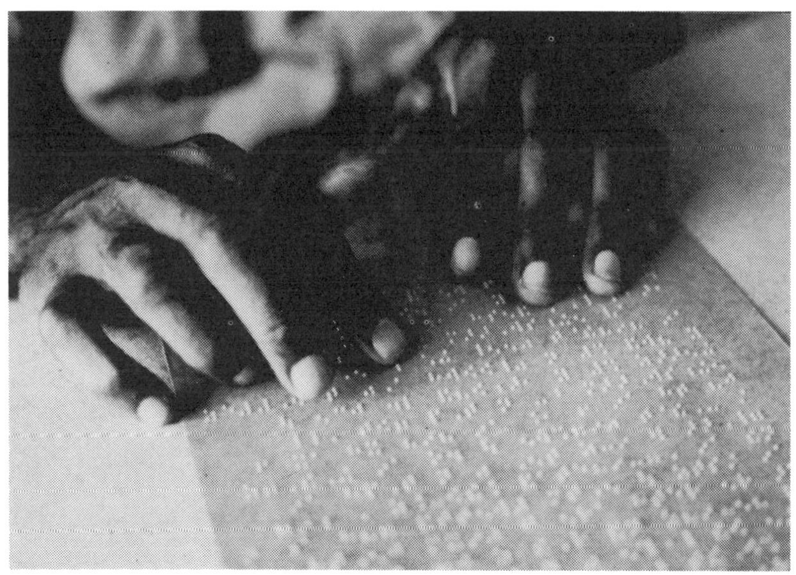

Hands glide over braille document.

learned to listen for those birds and to listen to his feelings deep inside. Arthur found he could have an insight without eyesight. He discovered that there were many others just like him. Arthur found they could love each other and learn to care no matter what their disabilities.

When the Lions League opened a three-month camp for crippled children and children with other handicaps in 1953, they did not realize that the "tiger they had by the tail" would become one of the foremost tigers in the world. The camp was to become the first Lions camp for the handicapped, one dedicated to helping a wide variety of people who had lost faith in themselves and hope for a rewarding life. Supported by the Lions of Texas and their friends, the camp for the children exceeded all expectations during the first four years. At this time the governing body for the camp, the Lions League, discussed putting together programs for the handicapped all year long.

So in 1958, the camp joined hands with the Texas Commission for the Blind and began a camp which was to operate as an adjustment training center for blind adults. Individuals accepted in the program were the newly blind and those who were beginning to lose their eyesight.

Arthur went to the Lions camp, and became one of the "tigers" at first. Soon he learned mobility in every kind of setting, from the rustic campsite to sidewalks in a busy city; he learned independent living skills and how to cope with a handicap. When he left the camp, he returned to his home in Houston with new confidence in himself and a willingness to establish a life in his community. He became a masseur, operated his own business and made as much as $160 a day profit. Arthur never forgot the Lions camp; he often called his old teachers there, and joked with them.

The blind program was discontinued in 1984, after having served more than 1,600 visually impaired individuals. It was made a part of the Texas Commission for the Blind's program in Austin, at their newly constructed Criss Cole Center. The camp went on to establish new programs so that the Lions of Texas would always follow their motto of "Our doors are never closed."

No history of the Texas Lions Camp would be complete without documenting the activities of the blind program during its twenty-six years duration at the camp. Its most important gift to the blind was assistance in helping them select a vocation with which they could become wage-earning, tax-paying citizens of their communities. The program was specifically built around the special needs of the trainees; it was, first and foremost, client-centered.

During this program, the Lions assisted men and women aged seventeen to ninety-five years, including those from all areas of life. They trained a young Spanish speaking girl from Del Rio who knew no English; another time they gave new "visions" to a highly professional middle-aged man who was one of the first atomic engineers for the U.S. government and in charge of NASA engineering for many years. He was Leo Zbanek, who had gone to Kerrville to "die" after losing his eyesight, but in Kerrville the Lions camp found him and persuaded him to enroll in their program. Zbanek decided he wanted to live. He said the Lions camp saved his life, so he joined the local Lions Club, became an enthusiastic worker for the camp and once more was a prominent leader in a community.

A participant during the early years of the Lions blind program was Nolan Underwood, who had been injured in an accident when he was fourteen. From his term at the camp, he went on to earn a B.A. degree in sociology and a masters in psychology. He returned to the camp to teach in the blind program for eight years and later became a public relations staffer and a licensed counselor for the camp on a permanent basis. In between, he was with the Texas Commission for the Blind, helped establish the Insight program for adult blind in San Antonio, was a counselor for the Kerrville State Hospital, was a private counselor to both children and adults, and worked with the University of Texas Health Science Center at San Antonio in individual and group therapy. Of great importance was that he had several operations and regained some of his eyesight after he had married, had three children and several grandchildren.

Underwood knew the desperate need of newly blind for survival. He said there were many newly blind who had responsibilities back home to support families. He said, "Here is where we see immediate results of our program." After personal adjustment training and renewed confidence, the head of a family sometimes went back home and returned to his same job.

Ruth Ann Harmon of Kerrville, blind from birth, entered the program and successfully began a new life for herself. She returned numerous years to sing for camp programs. Two girls from Guatemala took the course. They arrived in Houston hoping to find help. They did, as some Houston Lions had heard of them through a Lions network that encircled the globe in efforts to help people who had no means of helping themselves.

One year a man who had heard of the blind program called from New Orleans in an effort to get help for a friend who lived in Beirut. During the time the Lions clubs operated the blind program, persons came from over the world for the special attention. They remained in training for three to nine months, depending upon how soon they became mobile and were secure in their ability to resume their lives in a working community. The camp sometimes had day students, too; it was willing to take anyone who needed their help. Most stayed as residents for about three months.

It was not the camp's purpose to teach a profession to the blind participants. The focus was on assisting individuals in adjusting to their handicaps and developing skills necessary to function in day-to-day living with maximum independence. Among the general courses were daily living skills, mobility, communication, recreation, arts and crafts. Special classes included cooking, sewing, shopping, telephoning, money identification, typing, laundry,

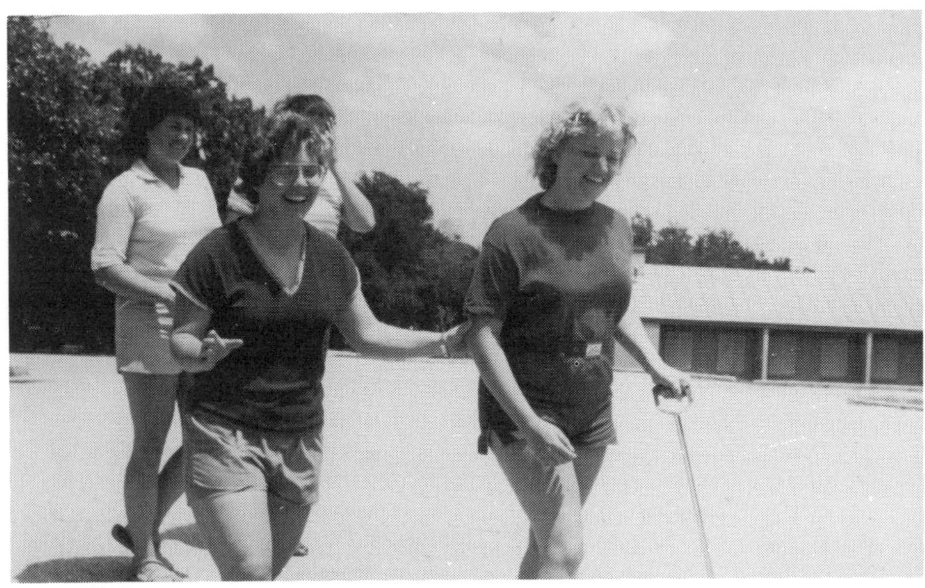

Learning mobility made fun in camp blind program.

home repair, job information, cane travel, braille writing, parties, bowling, pottery, and woodwork, personal grooming, personal hygiene, table etiquette, posture, dancing, and social games. Sometimes as many as seventeen men and women specialists were on the staff, but seldom were there more than thirty trainees. The center was proud of its small family atmosphere. Lions supporters considered the program a first step in guiding blind persons into the best field for a career and providing counseling for seeking specialized vocational training.

Instructors discovered early that the smooth paths on the campgrounds were designed for the physically handicapped children. They deliberately built hazards in certain places so that the blind students could practice with obstacles they might encounter in the "real" world. Just like the spirit of the summer camp for handicapped children, the winter program for the blind adults operated with a *can do* and optimistic attitude. Also, it was free of charge to all participants, with the Texas Commission paying part and the Lions organization paying the remainder.

When a trainee left the program, he was encouraged to help locate other possible trainees over the state. The Lions League wanted to provide as comprehensive and complete services to as many visually impaired people in Texas as they could. The Lions themselves helped to find blind persons needing training; and after a person completed the program, Lions were asked to work as follow-up volunteers, determining how well that person was adjusting and if he might need the Lions program again. Some did.

Central Texas communities became accustomed to being used as training grounds for the mobility classes. The trainees could be recognized by the white canes carried by all students. Teachers took them to Kerrville and other cities in the area to learn how to get around the streets and sidewalks, but the big one came when they were driven to San Antonio and taught to find their way safely and independently in a very crowded city.

Among the persons trained during the more than two decades of the blind program was a Lions member who, after completing the course, eagerly returned home, renewed old friendships and worked as a vital member of his Lions club. Traditionally, Lions clubs over the world have had special places in their service activities for assistance to the blind. They have transported thousands to doctors for needed attention and supplied more thousands with glasses to improve their vision.

A letter from a graduate trainee said: "The onset of blindness brought frustration, fear, and even humiliation. The training at the Lions camp corrected these misapprehensions, empowering me with confidence and a sense of can do. It even improved my sense of humor at accepting my own limitations. Overall, there was a climate of love and dedication which I could use in my attitude toward others. Thank you, Lions, for putting me back in business."

Since the Lions camp had plenty of room for all types of meetings, it leased its facilities throughout the winter months. For a number of years Region Thirteen Education Service Center held a four-day "baby camp" attended by parents and their babies or preschool children with vision problems. Focus of the camp experience was to provide families an opportunity to meet other parents with similar problems, experiences and solutions. Among topics addressed were sensory stimulation, motor development, language development, behavioral management, braille readiness, daily living, and communication and parental attitudinal concerns. Teachers certified in visually handicapped education were as-

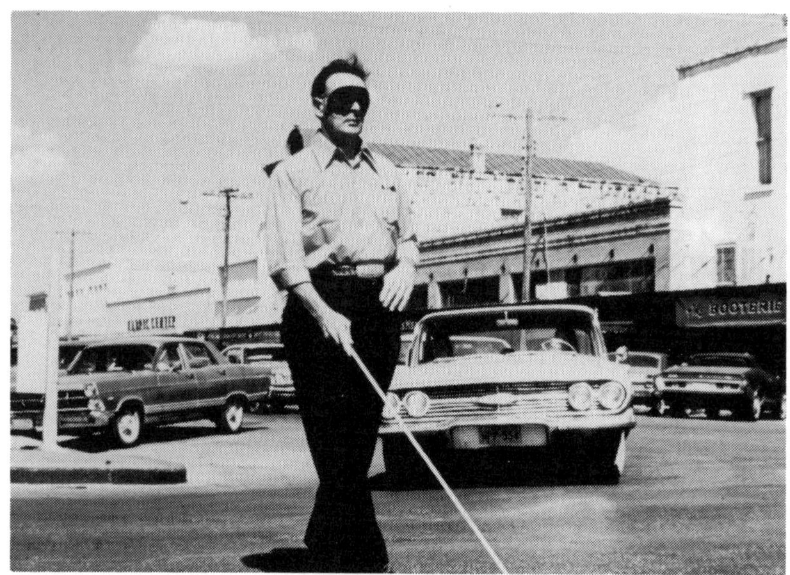

This man was almost at graduation point when he learned to navigate in crowded city areas.

sisted by others who were serving visually impaired infants and preschoolers.

Special education students from various universities served as babysitters while parents met together in classes. These workshops were funded as a pilot program by the Texas Education Agency free of charge. Among reasons the agency selected the Lions camp site was they had already had experience in their adult blind rehabilitation program and with visually handicapped children in summer camp. The Kerrville area, too, was centrally located for Texas parents served by all Education Service Centers.

When Glenn Crawford became executive director of the camp he was not a member of a Lions club. He was soon invited to affiliate, and he did. One day he was selling benefit tickets at a store in downtown Kerrville when a young woman walked up to him. A small baby was asleep on her shoulder. She gave him the money for a ticket, then refused it saying, "This baby is blind. I attended your blind baby classes, and I can never help the Lions as much as they helped me and my baby. Keep the ticket and use the money to help others." The mother used her newly gained knowledge to guide her child; she understood her own emotions as well. Crawford said that day he became more than a club member; "I became a *Lion.*" Later Crawford learned that the baby had grown to school age and was in a local elementary school. She developed along normal lines, as if she were a non-handicapped girl. Her I.Q. measured greater than 165; an I.Q. of 145 is considered genius level.

One graduating trainee said on leaving the hilltop camp, "This program has revitalized this tired body and mind. I'm worthwhile and can help myself and others."

— Chapter 15 —

"The Doors Are Always Open"

"We cannot measure this service in a material way because the greatest benefit of the camp is the hope and inspiration given to those who are our guests."

— Herb Petry, Jr., past president
Lions Clubs International

HISTORY OF TEXAS LIONS CAMP

1947–48

An idea for building a facility for handicapped children, who had no place to go to camp, became an obsessed dream for many Lions of Texas. The need for a recreation, rehabilitation and education facility was great because the state was in the midst of a polio epidemic which had left thousands of children to spend their lives in iron lungs and wheelchairs or on crutches. Leaders included men like Jack Roe of Kerrville and Jack Wiech of Brownsville.

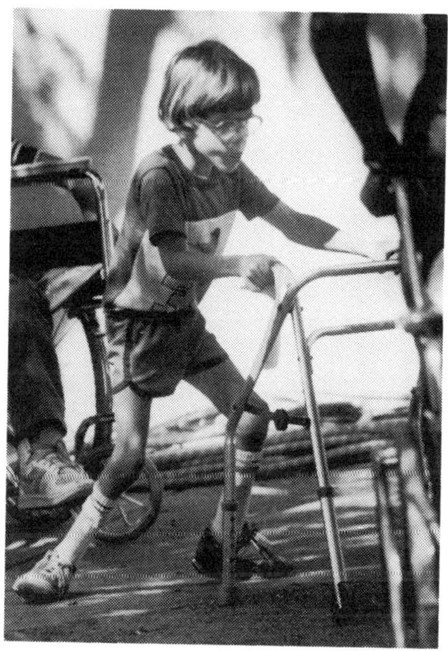

Campers find that determination pays off when conquering handicaps.

1949

Texas Lions League for Crippled Children, Inc., received charter from Texas Secretary of State as a tax-exempt, nonprofit corporation. Lions Clubs International voted approval of the camp to use its name and logo, the first known time this had occurred. Lion Wiech was elected first League president. Kerrville Lions Club discovered there was a beautiful hilltop parcel of 504 acres that might be available as a camp site from the federal government on a grant basis.

1950

After plowing through acres of red tape in Washington, D.C., the Lions League signed a sales agreement with the federal government. Acquiring permanent title to the land required the Lions League to raise $100,000 in six months. Dedicated Lions who supported the idea of the camp put thousands of miles on their automobiles, made hundreds of long distance telephone calls, spent hours writing letters and talking to other Lions. Governor Allan Shivers, a Lions club member, helped launch a statewide fund drive in a radio broadcast.

1951

Early in the year the Texas Lions raised the required $100,000. League directors approved a plan of one project per year per club to inject new life into the camp idea and voted to build two bunkhouses on the new camp site. Ground-breaking ceremonies were held in September with Secretary of State John Ben Sheppard as special guest, along with Past International Lions President Herb Petry, Jr., of Carrizo Springs.

Inhabitants of the enchanted 504 acres began to watch closely the strange activities going on in their world. Ol' Rusty, the big dark buck whose antlers were envied by all the other deer on the hilltop, could not explain the presence of the creatures tromping over the land on just two legs, waving their arms, talking in an unknown language. Rusty advised all animals on the hilltop to stay hidden in the woods, moving quietly and watching.

1952

The Lions League set June 1953 as opening date for the camp. Two bunkhouses, a dining room and kitchen, and an arts and crafts building for the camp were built. Bill Mickelsen was architect. The swimming pool was nearing completion, and the Houston Central and Gulf Coast Lions Clubs collected funds to build an infirmary. Wiech stepped down as League president, after serving the first four difficult years. Frank Robertson of San Antonio succeeded him. A. C. Jorns, well known photographer of Kerrville, began taking pictures every summer at the camp.

Ol' Rusty and all the animals kept close watch on camp activities. They could not understand why these funny creatures were bringing cut trees and other things to the hilltop, then making a lot of noise putting them together in strange ways. There were big things sprawled across what once was grazing land. But Rusty assured the animals that there were still enough woods for them to have their homes.

1953

June 8, forty boys and girls with various handicaps arrived at camp. There were eight counselors. The camp was officially dedicated on July 3. When summer was over the Lions facility had been

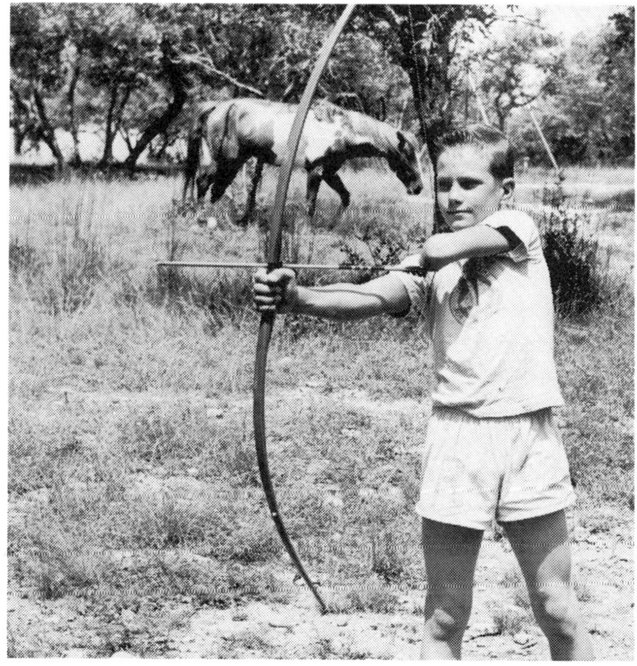

A camper in early days of Lions facility becomes skilled archer before his session ends.

host to 236 youngsters who found vitality and hope because of the things they learned at camp. The doors had been opened on the Lions special hilltop, and they would never close.

> *The raccoon family reported that the strange creatures were going into some parts of the woods, looking at plants and trees. Sometimes at night, they would sleep in the woods and gaze at the stars and moon. Ol' Rusty said he thought they meant no harm, but he believed the creatures meant to stay on the hilltop.*

1954

Texas Lions approved an annual dues-paying plan to give the camp financial stability. Two more bunkhouses had been completed, along with an administration building, the Jack B. Wright Memorial Chapel, and caretaker's cottage. Wright had been an outstanding member of the Founder Lions Club of San Antonio and worked hard for the camp. He said his life, outside of his family, had three parts — first, his duty to God; second, his help for handicapped children; and, this, his work in the Lions Club. The open-air chapel built on a hill by the San Antonio Lions in his memory, featured a huge, rough-hewn cross on the exterior which could be seen for miles around and by passing motorists on Highway 27. The chapel was formally dedicated, as well as the infirmary, and the campers had a part in both services. The new Lions Club of Ingram presented John Hill an honorary life membership in the camp for his work in preparing dirt pads for the bunkhouses and pathways for wheelchairs. He was just one of many Lions from throughout the state who contributed time, money, talents, or whatever they could to their camp for crippled children. Governor Shivers paid a visit to the camp, after which one camper, named Alfred Shivers, who was not a relative of the Texas official, was nicknamed "The Guvner."

1955

The campers loved arts and crafts so much that the building was expanded. Also a recreation hall was opened, and named for Frank Robertson, first executive director of the camp. A fifth bunkhouse was completed. The camp was exceeding all expectations. This was the third year that Randy had attended the camp, and he loved it. Because of polio his legs were weak and he was mobile only in a wheelchair, but in the swimming pool he was like a little fish. For three years he had wished he could jump off the diving board. A counselor carried him one day and placed him on the board. He crouched, steadying himself by his arms and hands, then crept forward and jumped! This was the year of Randy's great success and the year he decided he could do just about anything he wanted to do for the rest of his life.

Abilene Lions Club passed a memorial resolution to the late J. Clyde Penrod, a former president who was active in supporting the camp. When the camp was in a financial crises because of its building program, he launched his own fund-raising campaign. Penrod would take other Lions to the camp, pointing out its expanse of services and the needs for expansion. Many joined him in making large donations. However, he made a personal advance payment to the camp to enable the building to be completed.

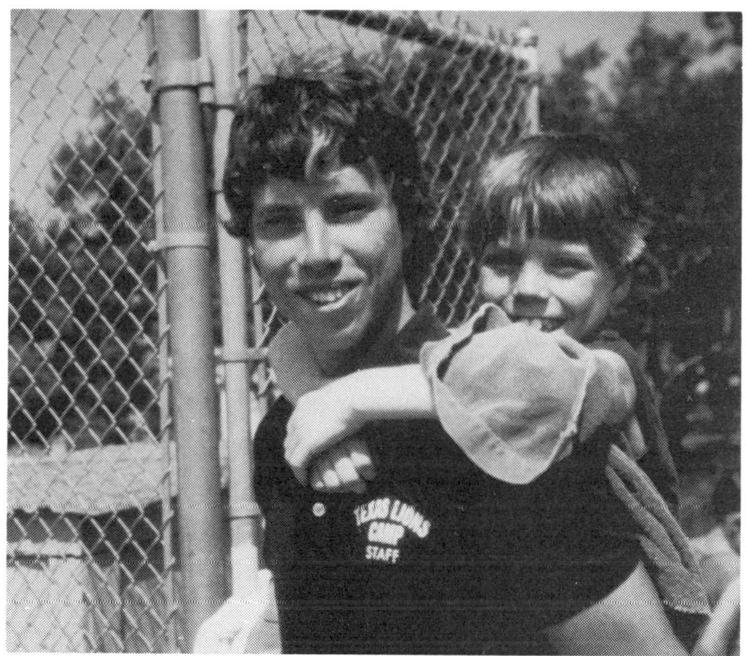

Bond between counselor and camper can be seen in happy faces.

1956

Lions found more children who wanted to come to camp. Word was spreading. A sixth bunkhouse was completed and camp enrollment reached an all-time high of 755 kids during the summer.

Ol' Rusty was gettin' old. He was still wise. He held a high-level meeting in the part of the woods not yet invaded by the strange creatures, who were becoming familiar to all the animals. None of the creatures ever bothered the animals or took away the things the animals needed to eat. Rusty's son, Swift, now had a little son, all legs and all spotted. One day the baby, whose name was Whisper, leaped too high and broke a thin, tender leg. Rusty and Swift had observed that some of the little creatures in the strange living places on the hilltop had legs that did not work very well. They took the baby to the edge of the woods where one of the big creatures found him. The creature carried the baby to his friends and they began doing things to his legs. They kept him a long time and patted him with love. Back in the woods, Rusty, Swift, and the baby's mother kept watch. Finally, after many nights had passed, the creatures brought the baby deer to the edge of the woods where he had been found. Whisper bounded into the bushes to find his fam-

ily. He was walking on the injured leg. He was jumping on the leg. Rusty asked every animal in the woods to be kind to the strange creatures. "They are here for a special purpose, and perhaps we can help each other."

1957

Camp was bulging at the seams. Lions over the state worked harder than ever to bring kids to camp and to supply funds for operation. The League received letters from over the nation, asking how to establish similar facilities. The original infirmary was converted to staff housing and program office, as a much larger staff was necessary. A new infirmary and a second staff house were constructed. League directors decided their facility could be used all year 'round, so they entered into an agreement with the Texas Commission for the Blind. The camp was to be used for nine months of the year to rehabilitate the newly blind and persons who were losing their eyesight.

1958

The adult blind program proved effective. Fifty-one trainees learned ways they could live more independently. The Lions dreams of helping those in need was truly unfolding in many ways on the central Texas hilltop. Janet, age nineteen, who had been blinded in an explosion, discovered that when she was sitting very still on Inspiration Point at night and listened very intently, she could see in her mind the night and the stars and the moon, and "almost heaven." She felt a new peace in her soul and a new joy in her heart. During summer camp, John, who was in leg braces, claimed to be the champion checker-player. Blind Doran challenged him. It took two hours of playing, and John was very surprised to end up on the short end of that contest.

1959

More children, more activities, more of everything was happening at the Lions camp. The recreation building was enlarged, and became a gymnasium for all kinds of programs. A garage was also added for storage. The camp was doing well financially, all year long now, and it had trucks and cars that waited to be placed in the new garage. Gordon, age seven, wanted to spend most of his

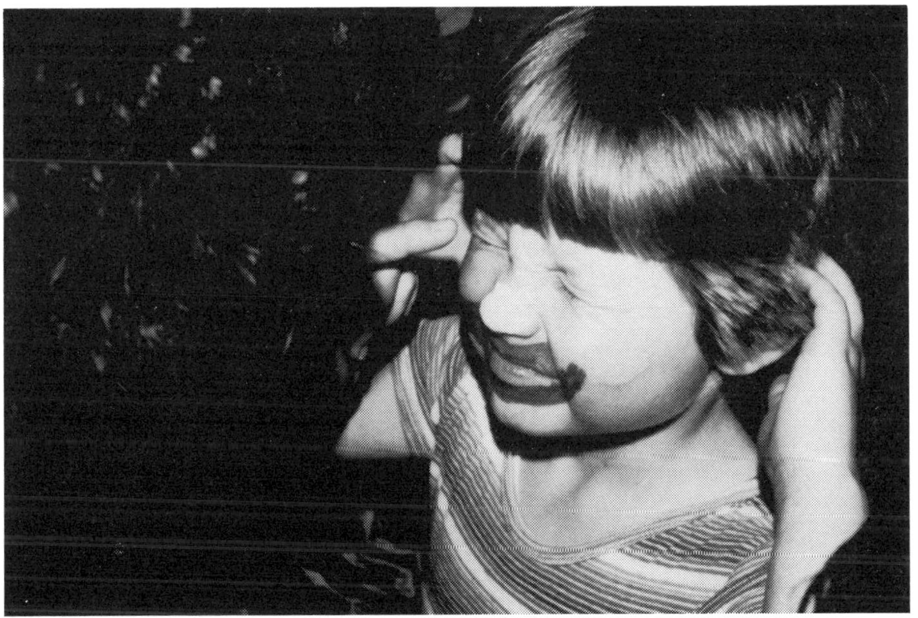

It is so much fun to get painted at carnival.

time in the arts and crafts building, because he discovered that he could use the two little hands that were attached to his shoulders. It took a long time, but he learned to plait tiny strips of leather. When he went home, for the first time in his life he gave his mother a present he had made, a plaited leather bracelet.

Both the Angleton and Temple Lions Clubs held minstrel shows to raise money for the camp. The Temple group called their show "Dixie Bell Jubilee." The Celeste Lions Club held their annual pancake supper and the Luling Lions sponsored Willard the Wizard and his magic show, both raising funds for the camp.

1960

This summer, 720 handicapped children found new courage at the Lions camp. Sixty-one blind trainees found new independence during the winter months.

The animals in the woods had come to accept all the strange things being done on their hilltop. They made their own special sounds every time they heard one of the creatures make a tinkling, merry sound. This happened all the time, and both the animals and the creatures felt happy about it.

A Cracker Jack sale was sponsored by the Paris Lions Club to raise camp money, while the Fairfield Lions challenged the Buffalo Lions in a basketball game. The winners were the children who attended the hilltop Lions camp.

1961

The camp played host to 721 youngsters during the summer, and sixty-three blind trainees in the winter. One of the campers, named Peg, whispered to a counselor next to her at the breakfast table. "See the counselor over there? The one in the purple shirt?" "Yes, what about her?" The inquisitive little Peg then asked, "Was she born that way?" "What way?" Actually, that particular counselor looked very normal. Then Peg queried: "Was she born with sign language?"

The recently organized Sinton Lions Club saw its first slides of the camp, after which they pledged to do their part to help keep the facility open and growing. Lions tailtwisters from the San Angelo Downtown and East Side Clubs held a "tailtwisters forum." April 14 was declared statewide Lions Candy Day when thousands of Texans sold candy door-to-door.

1962

Bill Smith, a non-Lion Texan, felt such concern for handicapped children he and his wife, Gladys, gave the camp enough money to build a duplex now used for staff lodging. The weekly TV show, "Route 66," came to the hilltop to film a special show, which excited everyone. This story had George Maharis, leading male star, becoming blind in an accident and going to the Lions blind rehabilitation program at the camp. He rescued a girl from the Guadalupe River, regaining his eyesight. During one camp session, the boys in Unit II drank thirty-eight bottles of milk to set a new record in milk-drinking. Janet learned to get in her wheelchair all by herself, and Ben spotted a rare Spanish Eagle's nest on a hill.

Brady Lions took a one-day trip to visit the camp, after which they challenged each other to greater service for their special children. Their tour guide at the camp was Eddie Parks Martin, who spent over thirty-five years as a counselor and public relations aide during summer camping.

1963

Texas Lions League for Crippled Children, Inc., looked back on its first successful decade, having been host to 6,455 handicapped children in the summers. During the winter, the adult blind trainees advanced to sixty-nine. At one of the camp sessions, Barbara won first place in the traditional pajama parade. She wore red PJs with feet in them. Since she was an amputee, she only needed one foot. She tied a big knot in the other pajama leg and hung a polka-dotted bow on it.

A fruit cake sale was the fund-raiser given by the Winnie- Stovall Club, and the Commerce Lions Club held a fund-raising chili feast at seventy-five cents for all a person could eat.

1964

Dedication of the William G. Davis Memorial Shelter, donated by Lions District 2T-3, was held. The large, open-air, roofed building provided a relaxed rest-stop in the middle of the camp. Lynn was in one of the camp sessions in 1964. She was long remembered for the many fruitful hours she spent learning to lace her shoes. "Snipe hunts" were popular. Daniel, suspected of having been on such a hunt before, told the new ones signed up that "it was fun. We chased it down the road and caught him in a sack. The poor little thing was scared, so we let it go."

Queen City Lions in Del Rio held a giant rummage sale to make money for the camp; Jasper Lions held a benefit rodeo; and Kilgore Lions sponsored a variety show and hootenanny at Kilgore College.

1965

Texas Lions Camp rocked along on a rosy course, growing and loving every minute of it. The staff, especially additional summer campers, needed housing. Pat and Ben Jackson donated money to build a beautiful dorm for blind women trainees in the winter program. His sister had been a trainee at the Lions center after she lost her eyesight. The large lodge was called the Jackson dorm and housed twenty eight persons. In one of the final camp sessions, David, age thirteen, became the crutch-balancing champion, and campers learned square dancing. The Navasota Lions Club held a spectacular Gay 90's Revue during which Lion and Mrs. Donald Kubricht rode a bicycle built for two.

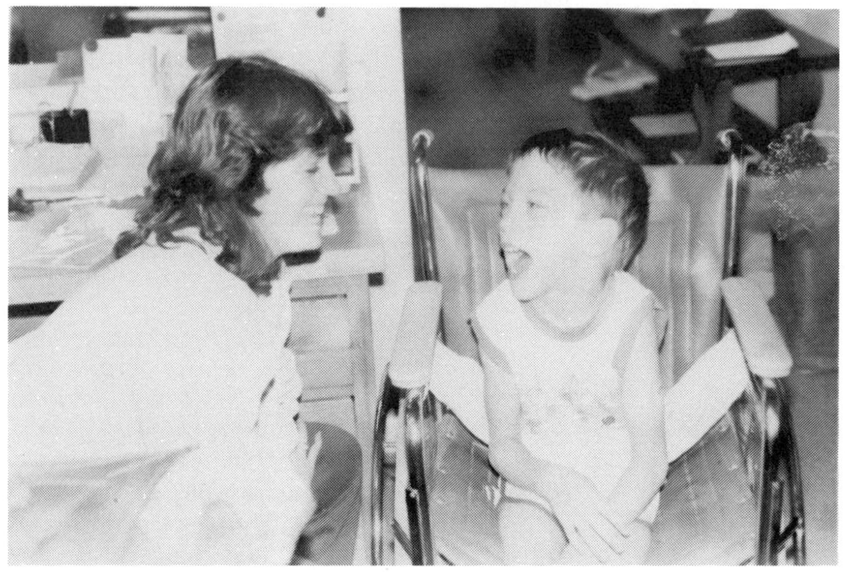

One of the best things to share is a laugh.

1966

This summer there were 750 children at the camp. As usual, many of the fun activities required some waiting in line. Shelley, a camper with a vision impairment, remarked one morning as he stood in line for breakfast, "Joann is lucky, she can wait sitting in her wheelchair. I have to sit standing up."

Friona Lions Club proudly counted a total of fifteen projects which they had sponsored for the camp in only five years.

1967

This summer was unusually hot for the Texas Hill Country, but most Lions campers complained little. The colorful country and customs of neighboring Mexico formed themes of most sessions. One small girl, wearing heavy braces on her legs, said seriously to a counselor, "I wish I was a Mexican." "Why?" asked the counselor. "Because then I would be able to speak Spanish." To which the counselor answered, "But you don't have to be Mexican to learn how to speak Spanish." "But what is the point in speaking

Spanish if I'm not a Mexican?" One unit was making Mexican pinatas. A little camper with cerebral palsy remarked as she attempted to glue crepe paper onto balloons, "I ate a pinata before but I never made one."

New Braunfels residents, Beth Elliott and Grace Foster, were presenting an increasingly popular musical in central Texas entitled "One Big Happy Family." One-half of all proceeds went to the Lions camp when several Lions clubs sponsored a series of one-nighters across the state.

1968

This year's figures for the hilltop program participants were 742 summer campers, and seventy-three blind trainees. Deer had become so accustomed to living with the strange two-footed creatures that many times they didn't bother to hide. George was on the hiking trail late one afternoon when he saw a small deer. It stood very still. "That deer is winking at me," he yelled. The next thing he saw was the white tail flicking up as it ran away.

1969

Swimming remained the most popular activity at the Lions camp. This year's attendance set a record, with 762 boys and girls in the summer, and eighty-four in the winter blind program. Maria was swimming in the shallow end of the pool. A chain link fence divided this area from the deep end of the pool. The fence was open on this afternoon, and Maria called, "You better close the gate; all the water is going to get out!"

1970

By the summer of 1970, the League had constructed an addition to the dining hall and expanded Bunkhouses I, II, and III. A nine-year-old boy named Jake came to camp. He had never fed himself, as his arms and hands were malformed and had little muscle coordination. Every member of his unit took turns trying to devise a way he would be able to feed himself. They were persistent, and it paid off. He was motivated, trying very hard, and by the second week he could manage almost an entire meal, depending on what was served. It was a turning point in Jake's life. Travis, who was a polio victim, arrived at camp very discouraged. He had

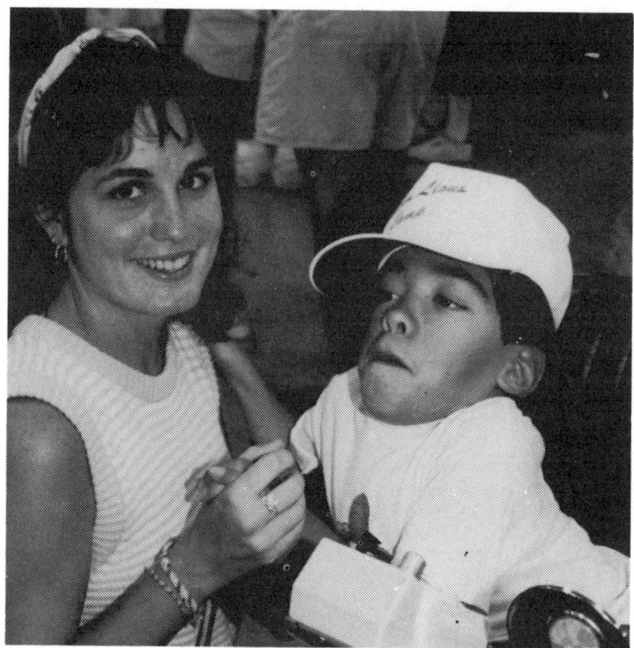

Counselor and camper dance at a party.

abandoned his physical therapy classes at home. When he saw all the kids swimming, he wanted to learn; and he did. He resumed his physical therapy when he returned home because he said he needed to stay in condition for swimming at camp next summer.

1971

This was a landmark year. The Lions of Texas added a new dimension of service to handicapped children by opening a pilot program for 111 diabetic campers on leased facilities at Friendswood, near Houston. Gabriel Ayub, Sr., who had been a Lion in Mexico, died in December. He had appealed to his sons to join some kind of service organization. Gabriel Ayub, Jr., joined a Lions Club in El Paso a few months before his father died, and Carlos Ayub joined the Lions in that same city ten days after his father's funeral. In the fortieth year of the Lions Camp, 1989, Carlos was a hard-working director of the League.

The chili supper held as a fund-raiser by the Pasadena Lions Club featured homemade root beer.

1972

Camp for the diabetic children was a dramatic success. Some 150 of them went to camp in 1972. One day the boys of one unit returned to camp with flowers for all the girls in their "sister" unit. Somehow Jenny, a counselor, did not receive a flower. "What about me," she called to the boys. "Don't I get any flowers." One of the girls answered, "Oh, Jenny, you don't need flowers; you have us and we don't wilt."

An article in the *Pampa News* said the Pampa Evening Lions Club was "lighting the city" by selling light bulbs door- to-door to help the children's camp. Pampa Noon Lions members held a musical program which introduced a premier act by three unnamed Lions, "Internationally Known Whistlers."

1973

Another all-time high in camp attendance came, with 1,058 handicapped boys and girls. Pete played the part of a peg-leg pirate during stunt night, and his portrayal was fairly easy. With the loss of one leg, all he had to do was attach what resembled a "peg" and cover an eye with a patch. One unit had trouble with seven-year-old Gary, blind from birth, who was always getting in someone else's bed.

Over 1,500 persons attended the Lubbock Lions Club beauty pageant, "Blossoming Queens from the Tea House of the Honorable Lions." Over 3,500 were said to have attended the Longview Lions Club barbecue and fiesta held on the Gregg County Fairgrounds.

1974

"Miracles of water" continued at the Lions hilltop camp, where many children found that here their handicaps were washed away. Donna, who had muscular dystrophy, was so excited when she found she could stand in water, she spent over an hour in the water with her counselor. "This is the first time I have ever stood up. Wait until my mother hears about it!" Her golden days continued; and by the end of camp, she was bobbing up and down alone and had achieved her first real victory in life.

1975

Number of campers served by the Lions this year totaled 1,019. Theme for the summer sessions was "Tropical Isle of Holidays," so the camp was continuously redecorated from snowy Christmas to Thanksgiving, July Fourth, Easter, and other special occasions. New facilities added included three tennis courts, a badminton court, golf driving range, new rooms on the infirmary and administration office, storage shelter at the lake and new garages. Robertson retired as executive director and J. L. McPherson assumed the position.

This year marked the thirty-fifth birthday of camp supporters, the Liberty Lions, and the Wills Point Club was founded.

1976

Number of handicapped children at summer camp was 724, while 310 diabetic children were served in two sessions. Julianna was a whisp of a thing who stayed quietly curled up in her wheelchair, always with a smile on her face. Counselors found her anxious to attend every activity, only to watch. At the overnight excitement on Inspiration Point Julianna remained quietly watching. The night was dark and the sky was filled with its special diamonds. It was time to stargaze. Suddenly Julianna's small voice burst forth, reciting stories of the planets, explaining about "light years away," and telling details of astronomy. Her place among her peers had been found high on a breezy hill.

1977

Texas Lions Camp was twenty-five years old. The dining hall was remodeled, the kitchen enlarged, a new water storage tank erected, and all electrical wiring placed underground. The League's figures indicated that 17,739 handicapped children had come through the gates. Some 1,247 blind adults had received rehabilitation training. The camp held an envious and prestigious position on an international scale. Highlight of the summer for campers was feeding and loving a baby rabbit which they named Fannie.

A summer camper was Allen, a teen-ager who had been a gridiron star and a tennis champion. Doctors discovered he had fibro sarcoma, a muscle cancer, on one thigh, so he was very depressed,

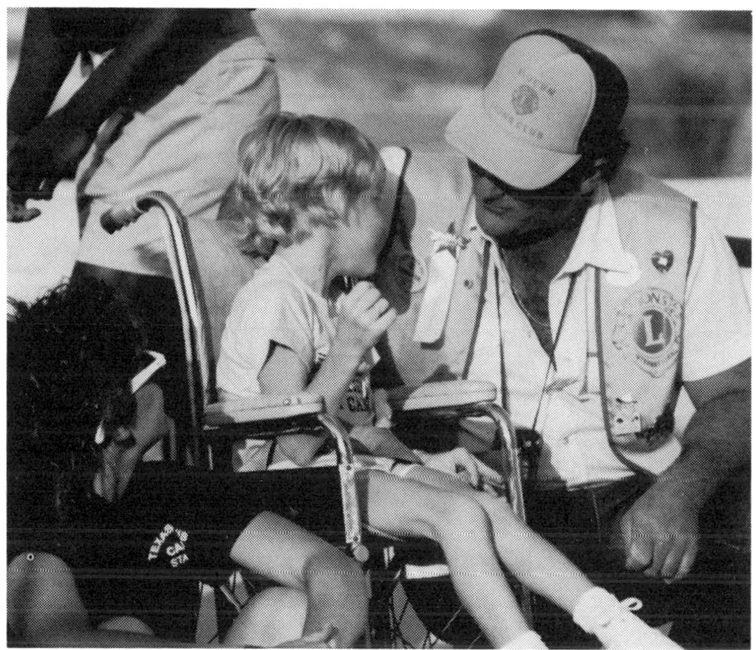

Lion member talks with young camper.

thinking he could no longer be an active athlete. Allen became too weak to run, but found he was still an athlete, this time as a champion swimmer.

1978

Glenn Crawford replaced J. L. McPherson, who retired as executive director of the camp. Victor Real Estate gave funds for a resident hall, and furnishings were provided by donations from Texas Lions clubs and their friends. Additional pews and concrete walks were added to the chapel.

1979

A new playground was constructed, the program office was renovated, and more applications came in than could ever be assigned in one summer. A youngster woke up at home one morning to find he couldn't move, and he spent months in respiration therapy. He felt that life had simply passed him by and that there would be no more baseball or football. He came to camp one year and put his life back together. Today he is president of a holding company for a Dallas bank.

The Mineola Lions Club held its first annual Wood County Fall Gun and Knife Show to benefit the camp; and five Lions clubs from Breckenridge, Cisco, Ranger, Moran, and Strawn, sponsored a benefit football game between Ranger and Cisco Colleges.

1980

Diabetic camping at Friendswood was discontinued by the Lions who brought these children to the Hill Country. One session was held at the camp and one session at nearby Camp Rio Vista. The League set up a goal of $550,000 for Phase I of a much needed expansion. A gazebo picnic area was constructed and a stone rail fence was built at the camp's entrance. During one summer session Burns Taylor brought his violin and was the most popular boy at camp, and Counselor Van taught Jimmy, who was visually impaired, to use a cane which opened new avenues for mobility for the teen-ager.

1981

Phase I was successfully completed, and visitors and campers saw two new bunkhouses, a second swimming pool, a remodeled kitchen, a pool patio, and upgraded utility equipment. During a summer softball game the two camper teams were tied eight to eight. With two outs and a man on first, the batter swung and hit a ground ball between first and second, hitting the base runner. The runner stopped, bent over and picked up the ball. He began jumping for joy, yelling, "I have the ball, I have the ball." All of a sudden he turned to the counselor in confusion, sadly asking "Does this mean the game is over?" The counselor answered, "Yes, but you are not a loser! Everybody at the Texas Lions Camp is a winner."

1982

Navy Seabees from Beeville, came to the hilltop and built a campcraft log cabin with a porch, and then prepared a road and parking lot area for paving. Clint Bench, thirteen, won a number of honors at camp, then went home to tell the Mineral Wells Evening Lions Club, his sponsor, what it was like to be a camper on that special hilltop. He received a high honor when the staff asked him to return next summer as a counselor-in- training, and the Mineral Wells Lions were very proud of their camper. Lionesses about the state sold large Christmas coloring books to make money for the camp.

1983

The Texas Lions Camp, as well as every facet of its operation and support over the state, took on a professional aura and surged upward in growth. The board attributed this to Glenn Crawford's guidance, including his selection of the best personnel available. Construction of the Herb Petry Sports Center began. This was the large area where there were soccer and baseball fields, exercise paths with therapeutic instructions, fountains and restrooms, and tennis courts. Alice McCreless gave needed exercise equipment in honor of her Lion husband, Sealy, a staunch, lifetime supporter of the camp. Renovation of the recreation hall also began; and a horse barn and corral were built. Members of the Midland Downtown Lions Club collected $3,000 for their camp fund at a Pancake Jamboree.

1984

The blind program was discontinued, as the Texas Commission for the Blind felt their new facilities in Austin could accommodate all persons being rehabilitated. The League opened its Outdoor Education Center to replace the blind project. Horseback riding had been enthusiastically welcomed, and both the corral and the riding arenas were expanded. Outdoor Education brought in enough money and staff to make having horses in the summertime feasible. Elena caught her first fish down at the pond and was proudly displaying it to other campers on the bank when it flopped off the hook. She let go her crutches to scramble after it. Splash! She fell back into the shallow water, but came up with her fish clutched tightly in both hands.

1985

Outdoor Education, a new concept, was exploding on the hilltop! During the year, 3,000 individuals participated, from after-school archaeological classes with hands-on lessons to week days

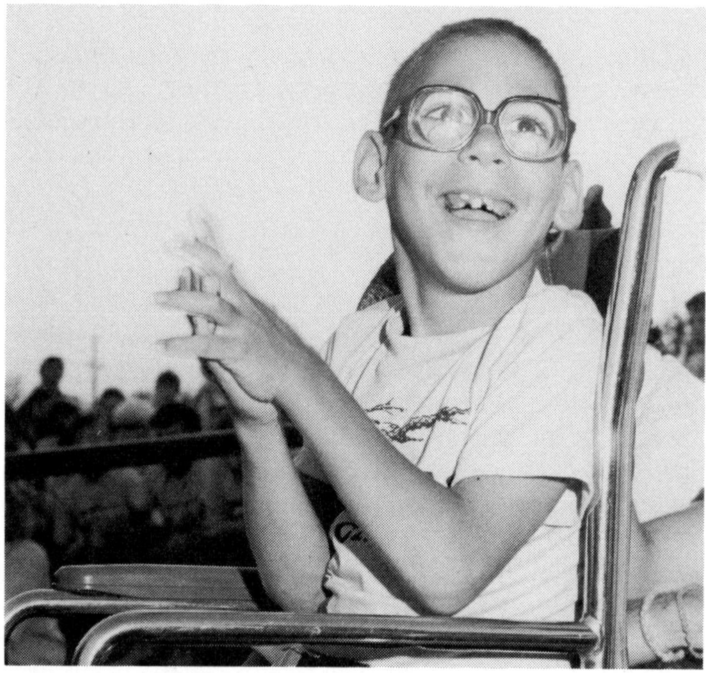

Success of Lions dream can be seen in the faces of their special children.

for blind children. The Lions OE Center was accredited as a private school by the Texas Education Agency, sending it into the field of recreational instruction as a leader. Other innovative additions included the therapeutic exercise trail, the Oak Cliff picnic area, and the Eagle nature trail with outdoor "classrooms." Video equipment was donated for the children's entertainment and for promotional purposes for the staff. "The Wizard of Oz" was the first video campers saw. The recreation hall/auditorium was renovated in time for the first camping session. Shelters for the riflery and archery ranges were built. The "new" amphitheater was completed, with a capacity of 600 persons. It was filled to capacity with campers and visitors the first awards night after completion.

1986

This marked the first year that the camp had facilities and staff to hold all diabetic sessions at the main campsite. The Outdoor Education Center became affiliated with the worldwide Elderhostel program, and several week-long Elderhostels were held during the winter months. Crawford said he met a former camper, who later became a counselor, while visiting his daughter at North Texas University in Denton. The former counselor explained that she would soon graduate with a degree in therapeutic recreation, a goal she picked while at camp. Belton Lions staged a benefit entitled "We Are The Weird," based on a satirical fund-raising campaign to relieve the world of stupidity. It *did* raise money for the children's camp.

1987

Texas economy hit a slump. This was the first year in Texas Lions history that children had to be turned away from camp. Distressed Lions over the state and other concerned groups planned benefits and tried to take measures so that never again would a handicapped child be turned away from the hilltop.

There seemed to be more deer, rabbits, and wildlife on the 504 acres than ever before.

Ol' Rusty died many years before, but each generation of deer heard the story of when the strange creatures came to their woods, and stayed. Ol' Rusty had once said that before the newest strange creatures there had been Indian creatures, who knew how to live with the animals and birds also. He felt that the Great Spirit must have sent the new creatures to replace the Indians, for they seemed to love the same things that Indians loved: animals and birds, campfires and coup feathers.

1988

One of the new summer activities was a rodeo, which included regular rodeo events plus fun contests on horses such as musical chairs and egg-in-the-spoon. This event was presented with a grand entry of horses, campers, counselors, volunteers, and spectators. With more horses and trained instructors, horseback riding was stressed, and campers looked forward to 1989 with enthusiasm to learning more sports centered around horses. In addition, therapeutic riding was taking an important place in the outdoor center schedules. The Santo Lions Club built a huge, metal-fenced arena for rodeos and horse shows. The camp planned to put up lights so horse events could be held later, and the League could rent out the large, modern facility to other groups. The well known TV show, "Eyes of Texas," devoted one of its programs to the Texas Lions Camp, and was seen by TV viewers all over the state.

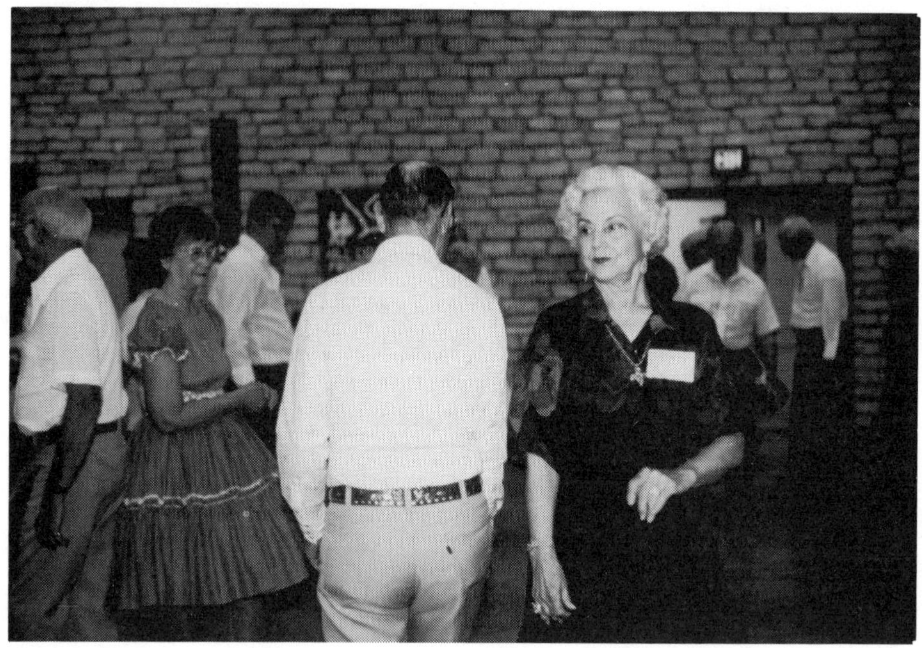

Elderhostel couples learn western dancing.

1989

The three facets of the Lions League was growing, including the camp for handicapped children, the camp for diabetic children, and the outdoor education center. There was talk of offering "Challenge Programs" for handicapped young people, including water skiing, snow skiing, and overnight horse packing trips. The curriculum manual for staff, first known to be developed in the world of camping, was expected to be used in college-credit courses in the future. The program staff was working to expand counselors' college credit for their work in the summer.

The camp continued to try to reach as many of the eligible 225,000 handicapped children in the state as possible. Forty years before when the Lions League had been set up to organize and operate the camp, there were 552 Lions clubs, 32,592 members, and eight districts in Texas; in 1989 there were 1,100 clubs, over 40,000 members, and sixteen districts. Cost of the first summer camp in 1953 was $250,000, and the site contained two bunkhouses, dining room and kitchen, an arts and crafts building, an infirmary, and a swimming pool. There were 236 campers that year, costing the

Lions $81 per camper. In 1988, there were eight bunkhouses, two swimming pools, and twenty-one other buildings on a large and developed campsite. That year 1,103 boys and girls went to camp, costing the Lions clubs $75 per day per handicapped camper and $134 per day per diabetic child. Many dreams were in the making. Camp Development Director Ron Anderson had worked three years to collect $400,000 from non-Lions — corporations, individuals, and foundations — for a needed new administration building. At the beginning of 1989 he had reached his goal. Some $50,000 of the goal, however, had come from the Lions Clubs International Foundation.

Texas Lions knew they could always count on a director/ tail-twister keeping funds and plans moving over the state and into the camp, Inspiration Point and Suddenly as overnight campsites, a counselor's shoulder to cry on, that certain "Spirit of Camp," the big Texas night sky, the aura of self-assurance and battles won, League presidents passing on the gavel, old buildings being torn down to make way for new ones, the excitement of awards night, the Friendship Circle about campfires, taps and reveille, tears when campers and counselors moved down the winding road and through the gate, saying goodbye.

Jack Roe, who was credited with having the idea for a camp for crippled children, said, "If the Lions of Texas never do another thing this camp will justify their rating as the largest organization of service clubs in the world."

Sharlette Haley, who was a waterfront counselor in 1985, wrote the following poem about the Texas Lions Camp

In a world filled with troubles and pain
In an age when wrong is right.
At a time when only a few seem to care
It is then that I begin my fight.

In this small place that I call home
It's the only real home I know
For it is here that all my troubles can die
And only true love can grow.

To touch the life of a small child in pain
To show the blind boy the way
To listen to the deaf girl when no one else will
To love them every day.

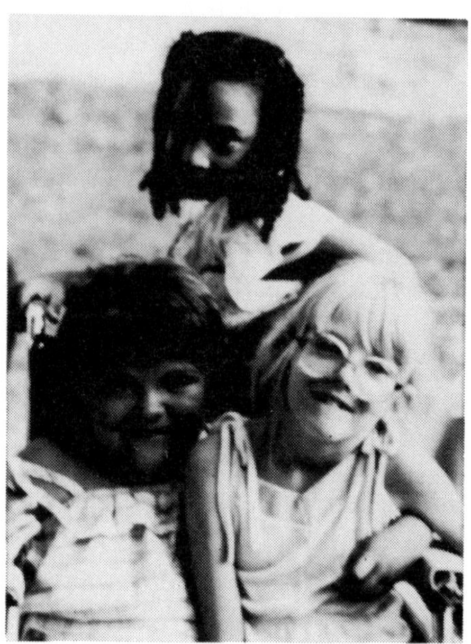

Best thing at camp is making friends with others who understood.

A small hug before she falls asleep
A tiny peck on his shaking hand
A reassuring nod when he's scared of the dark
The hurt only you understand.

The restroom trip at three in the morning.
That long, tiring push up the hill
Waiting patiently for her to walk down the road
Begging him to swallow his pill.

Dancing with him when he can barely stand
Encouraging him to catch those balls
Teaching her to hold her breath under water
And comforting her when she falls.

My life is dedicated to all of these tasks
Though tasks they don't seem to me
They are acts of love from my Heavenly Father
And I thank Him for giving them to me.

He placed in my heart a special love
That only He can help me to show
And I praise Him for giving me all my kids
So I can let that special love flow.

Index

A
Abilene Lions Club, 126, 166
Abilene, Texas, 126
Ackerman, Lou, 93
Administration of General Services, 12
Akridge, J. L., 108
Alamo Heights Lions Club (San Antonio), 145
Alice Lions Club, 125
Alvin Lions Club, 126
American Camping Association, 38, 64, 144
American Diabetes Association, 64
American Legion, 5
American Red Cross, 38, 140
Anderson, Ronald "Ron" Ray, 95, 124, 126, 136, 143, 144, 147, 183
Andrysiak, Thomas, 46, 145, 147
Angleton Lions Club, 169
Arnold, Betty, 145
  Bonnie, 69
  Erich, 145
Ashwood, Toni, 145
Atkins, Brian, 145
  Dean, 145
Augusta, Michigan, 100
Austin, Texas, 13
Awards Night, 46–47, 48
Ayub, Carlos, 174
  Gabriel, Jr., 174
  Gabriel, Sr., 174

B
Barnes, Don, 143, 144, 146
  Linda, 145
Barsh, Herbert F., 108
Beaser, Mr., 10
Bellaire Lions Club, 126
Belton Lions Club, 181
Benbrook Lions of Fort Worth, 126
Bench, Clint, 178
Bombeck, Erma, 137
Bowman, Rick, 126
Brabham, Rev. Tom, 3
Brady Lions Club, 170
Breckenridge Lions Club, 178
Brown, George, 10, 18
  Houriah, 30
  Joshua, 5
Brownsville Downtown Lions Club, 127
Brownsville, Texas, 4
Buffalo Lions Club, 170
Butt, Howard, 21

C
Camp Horsemanship Association, 100
Camp Manison (Friendswood), 64–65
Camp Olympia (Houston), 90
Camp Rio Vista (Ingram), 67, 178
Carter, Elizabeth, 30
Catholic Standard, 86
Caves, Gary, 90
Celeste Lions Club, 169
Century Club, 109
Charles Schreiner Company, 136
Children's Diabetes Management Center, 65
Children's Division, Federal Security Administration, 10
Childress Lions Club, 127
Church, R. G., 10
Cisco College, 178

Cisco Lions Club, 178
Clark, Tom, 11
Clarke, Bobby, 71
Colorado State University, 144
Commerce Lions Club, 171
Connally, John, 8, 10
  Tom, 10
Conroe Lions Club, 109
Cooke, Bill, 128
Cooper, Marshall, 7, 108
Council of Governors of Texas, 4
Cox, Dr. George, 8
Crawford, Glenn, 20, 36, 47, 54, 57, 67, 68, 70, 72, 78, 90, 95, 96, 100, 106, 108, 111, 122, 124, 128, 136, 141, 142, 143, 144, 145, 147, 149, 160–161, 177, 179
  M. A., 145, 148
Creswell, Shirley, 30
Criss Cole Center, 156
Crockett, J. L., 33
Cross, Joann, 97
Cypress Trail U.M.C. Children's Choir (Spring), 135

D

Daeschner, Dr. C. W., 65
Dallas, Texas, 12, 13, 14
Davis, Roy N., 108
Dean, Nelda, 145
DeWitt, W. C., 135
diabetes, 60–73
Dickerson, Windell, 32
Division of School Administration, 12
Doc, 31
Dollins, Betty, 28
Dr. Salk, 1
Driskill, W. E. (Pete), 17
Duchene, Roberto, 31
Dudley, Lu, 104
Dusold, Dr. Richard, 68

E

Eagle Aerie, 133
Education Service Center, 159, 160
Elderhostels, 92, 95, 96, 141, 180
Elliott, Beth, 173

F

Fairfield Lions Club, 170
Family Learning Vacation, 96
Federal Security Agency, 8, 11, 12, 17
Field Newspaper Syndicate, 137
Fisher, Marlowe C., 8, 10, 11
  O. C., 8, 33
Follett Educational Corporation, 144
Fort Worth Lions Club, 33
Foster, Grace, 173
Founder Lions Club (San Antonio), 165
4-H Clubs (Kerrville), 134
4-H Youth Programs, 92
Fraternal Order of Eagles, 133
Friendship Circle, 44, 47, 58, 112, 183
Friendswood, Texas, 67, 178
Friona Lions Club, 172

G

Gallegos, Diego, 33
Galloway, Victor, 92
Garcia, Fabian, 145
Geiger, James, 29
General Services, 12
Gentry, George, 10
  George P., 18
Gleckler, Jacqueline, 29, 31, 33
Gore, Bobby, 145
Grace, Jennifer, 145
Graham Noon Lions Club, 128
Green, Joy, 30
Gregg County Fairgrounds, 175
Grindstaff, E. J., 108
Guadalupe River, 5, 9, 170
Gulf Coast Lions Club, 20

H

Haley, Sharlette, 183
Hamilton, Fred, 108
  Street, 22
Haren, Joe, 145, 148, 149
  Judy, 148
Harmon, Ruth Ann, 157
Harris, Sid, 6
Havor, June, 32
Hawkins, Tyrus, 30
Hayes, Tim, 144–145
Hays, Louis, 30
Heart O' The Hills, 127
Herb Petry Sports Center, 179
Heritage Creative Outdoor Advertising Company, 135
Hielscher, C. N., 33

Hill, John, 166
Hill Country Arts Foundation's Point Theatre Box Office (Ingram), 135
Hill Country Charity Ball Association, 133–134
Holcomb, Greg, 101, 145
horseback riding, 99–103
Host Lions Clubs (Kerrville), 127
Houston Central Lions Club, 20
Houston Fat Stock Show, 134
Houston and Gulf Coast Diabetes Association, 65
Houston, Texas, 16, 154, 156
Hudson, Wilma, 145
Hunt, Mark, 145
Hurricane Gilbert, 140
Hyer, Julien C., 3, 11, 130

I

Independent School District (Temple), 144
Industry West-End Lions, 128
Inspiration Point, 20, 29, 31, 44, 111, 112, 149, 168, 176
International Association of Lions Clubs (New York City), 4
Itz, Marilyn, 30

J

Jack B. Wright Memorial Chapel, 165
Jacksboro Lions, 128
Jackson, Ben, 133, 171
  Pat, 4, 107, 171
Jackson Dormitory/Lodge, 133
Jasper Lions Club, 171
Johnson, Lyndon B., 8, 9, 10, 12
Jones, Dan, 32
  Melvin, 4, 111
Jordan, George R., 14, 129
  Roland C., 108
Jorns, A. C., 164

K

Kegin, Debbe, 145
Kennedy, Theo Ann, 30
Kerrville Catholic Church, 57
Kerrville Daily Times, 69, 76
Kerrville Lions Club, 3, 126, 163
Kerrville State Hospital, 157
Kerrville, Texas, 2, 5, 7, 11, 12, 13, 15, 22, 33, 49, 51, 67
Kester, Joan, 29, 30
Kilgore College, 171
Kilgore Lions Club, 171
Killeen Lioness Club, 128
Kirby, Dann, 148
  Harriette, 148
Koennecke Scholarship Award, 85
Kubricht, Mr. and Mrs. Donald, 171

L

Lackey, Mike, 92, 145
LaFours, 135
Lake Brownwood Lioness Club, 128
Laredo Evening Lions, 127
League Directors, 113–121
Liberty Lions Club, 176
Lione, 31, 33
Lions Candy Day, 170
Lions Club (Ingram), 166
Lions Clubs International, 4, 11, 13, 163, 185
Lions Clubs International Convention (Toronto), 129
Lions Clubs International Foundation, 183
Lions International, 16
Livingston, Texas, 126
Longhorn Recreation Lab, 92
Longview Lions Club, 175
Lopez, Oscar, 74, 78, 80–82, 124, 145
Lubbock Lions Club, 127, 175
Luling Lions Club, 169

M

Mac, 31
MacKaron, Phil, 76
McCracken, J. P., 108
McCreless, Alice, 179
  Sealy, 15, 179
McDonalds (Galveston), 135
McGonagill, George, 148
McLaughlin, E. Ray, 108
McMurray College, 126
McPherson, J. L., 108, 145, 176, 177
Maharis, George, 170
Mahon, Marie, 30
Martin, Eddie Parks, 84, 170
Martinez, Jane, 30
Mayer, E. B. (Tex), 16

Memorial Lions Club (Houston), 125
Mickelsen, Bill, 6, 7, 8, 10, 11, 13, 17, 19–20, 164
Midland Downtown Lions Club, 179
Minear, Virgil, 4, 107
Mineola Lions Club, 178
Mineral Wells Evening Lions Club, 178–179
Monahans Lions, 128
Moore, J. I., 2, 4, 107, 136
  Mary Tyler, 71
Moran Lions Club, 178
Moss, Anna, 30
Munger, E. H., 108
Murray, Buddy, 147
  J. C. "Buddy," 13, 30
  Vera, 147

N

National Conference of Lions Camps, 92
National Foundation for Infantile Paralysis, 53
National Milk Bowl, 135
Navasota Lions Club, 171
New Braunfels Noon Lions Club, 126
Newell, Jodi, 145
Newman, Mildred, 22
New York City, NY, 144
Nickelson, Randy W., 129, 130
North American Handicapped Riding Association, 100
Notre Dame Catholic School, 134

O

Office of Surplus Real Estate, Public Building Administration, 10
O'Quinn, Chris, 93, 94, 95, 96, 145
Outdoor Education Center, 95, 142, 179, 180 (*see* Texas Lions Camp Education Center)
Outdoor Education Program, 91

P

Pakan, Sam, 108
Pampa Evening Lions Club, 175
Pampa News, 175
Paris Lions Club, 170
Pasadena Lions Club, 174
Paul, George, 125
Penrod, J. Clyde, 166
Perry, Arthur C., 10
Peterson, Hal, 22
Petry, Herb, 11, 13, 18, 33, 185
  Herb, Jr., 164
Pipkin, Maurice, 20
Price, R. E., 108
Project Wild Curriculums, 92
Pruneda, Carolina, 145

Q

Queen City Lions (Del Rio), 171
Queen of Great Britain, 129

R

Ramsey, F. A., 8
Ranger College, 178
Ranger Lions Club, 178
Real, Victor, 133
Real Lodge, 133
Real Property Disposal of the General Services, 12
Reichle, Gene, 29
Reporter, 128
Rhymes, Mae Nell, 145
Riley, Schley, 4, 107
Rio Grande Valley, 134
Robertson, Frank, 18, 19, 21, 22, 27, 29, 33, 108, 145, 164, 166, 176
  Mr., 31
Robinson, Effie, 110, 136, 137
  W. L., 110, 136
Rockdale Noon Lions Club, 128
Roe, Jack, 2, 3, 7, 10, 18, 21, 30–31, 34, 145, 162, 183
  Linn, 30
Roper, John, 144
Rowan, Dan, 71
Rowlett Lions Club, 109
Ruth, A. J., 135
Rutherford, W. R., 4, 107

S

Salk, 63
Sample, Earline, 30
San Angelo Downtown Lions Club, 170
San Angelo East Side Lions Club, 170
San Antonio Lions, 166
San Antonio, Texas, 125
Santo, Ron, 71
Santo Lions Club, 100, 181

Schreiner College, 127
Schreiner family, 5
Scott, Sue, 30
Shaffer, Walt, 16, 17
Shaw, Barbara, 30
Sheppard, John Ben, 18, 164
Shivers, Alfred, 166
  Allan, 10, 13, 18, 164, 166
Shrine's Crippled Children's Hospital, 14
Singer Corporation, 144
Sinton Lions Club, 170
Smith, Bill, 170
  Gladys, 170
  Keith, 99, 100, 102, 145
  Reagan, 4, 18, 107, 108
Soboslay, Marilyn, 30
Southard, Rand, 35, 38, 41, 78, 143, 144, 145
Southern Methodist University (Dallas), 144
Southern Methodist University (San Antonio), 144
South Texas Regional Deaf Educators Conference, 92
Southwest Conference, 135
Southwest Texas State University, 144
Spears, Adrian A., 10
Spivey, J. Harold, 147
Stephen F. Austin University (Nacogdoches), 144
Stobaugh, Earl, 29
Stone, Dick, 30
Stonewall, Texas, 134
Stovenour, Bobby, 32
Strawn Lions Club, 178
Suddenly, 44
Surplus Property Utilization Program, 12
Sylestine, Terry, 84

T

tailtwisters, 105–122
Talbert, Billy, 71
Taylor, Burns, 178
Temple Lions Club, 169
Texas Agricultural Extension, 92
Texas Basketball Festival (Kerrville), 126
Texas Center for the Blind (Kerrville), 154
Texas City Lions Club, 16, 17
Texas Commission for the Blind, 154, 155, 168
Texas Commission for the Blind (Austin), 156, 179
Texas Departments of Public Welfare, Rehabilitation and Health, 3
Texas Education Agency, 34, 90, 94, 160, 180
Texas Health Department, 8
Texas Lions Camp for Crippled Children (Kerrville), 28
Texas Lions Camp Education Center, 92–97
Texas Lions convention (San Angelo), 4
Texas Lions League camp, 22–24
Texas Lions League for Crippled Children, Inc., 171
Texas Parks and Wildlife Department, 130, 134–135, 144
Texas School for the Deaf, 92
Texas Science Teachers Association, 92
Texas Secretary of State, 4, 163
Texas Southmost College, 20
The Crutch, 31
therapeutic riding, 99
Tivy High School, 127
Toops, Eleanor, 143, 144
Travis, Dr. Luther B., 65, 70–72
Two Sisters Antiques (Kerrville), 135

U

U.S. Attorney General, 10
U.S. Commissioner of Education, 12
U.S. Navy Seabees (Beeville), 135, 178
U.S. Public Health Service, 8
Underwood, Nolan, 95, 126, 144, 147, 156, 157
  Peggy, 145
University of North Texas, 142
University of Texas, 95, 144
University of Texas Health Science Center (San Antonio), 157
University of Texas Medical Branch (Houston), 65

V
Vansch, A. D., 10
Vaughn, Mr., 31
Veterans' Hospital, 57
Victor Real Estate, 177

W
W.R. Grace Educational Products, 144
Waco News-Tribune, 28
Waifs and Strays Society, 129
Waller, Jim Ed, 108
Ward, James, 108
Warden, C. W. (Chuck), 135
Warren, Buda, 30
  Fanny, 30
Washington, DC, 6, 10, 11, 12, 86
Weslaco Lioness Club, 125
Wheeler, James H., Jr., 108
White, Raymond, 108
White Oak, Texas, 147
Wiech, Jack, 2, 3, 4, 5, 6, 7, 8, 9, 10, 11, 12, 13, 17, 18, 19, 27, 33, 107, 108, 127, 129, 162, 163, 164
William G. Davis Memorial Shelter, 171
Williams, J. E., 10
Wills Point Lions Club, 176
Winnie-Stovall Club, 171
Woodard, Wilbert, 29
Wood County Fall Gun and Knife Show, 178
Wright, Jack B., 33
Wright Memorial Chapel, 44

Z
Zbanek, Leo, 156
Zimmermann, Jerry, 30